D1456672

Why Do I Feel So Lousy?

How to lose weight, lower cholesterol and triglyceride levels, eliminate migraines and digestive problems, slow down aging and just plain feel better!

by

Lorrie Medford, C.N.

LDN Publishing
P.O. Box 54007
Tulsa, Oklahoma 74155

WHY DO I FEEL SO LOUSY?
How to lose weight, lower cholesterol and triglyceride levels, eliminate migraines and digestive problems, slow down aging and just plain feel better!

ISBN #978-0-9676419-6-6
Copyright © 2003 Lorrie Medford, C.N.
LDN Publishing
P. O. Box 54007
Tulsa, OK 74155

Library of Congress Cataloging-in-Publishing Data

Medford, Lorrie

      Why Do I Feel So Lousy?
      Lorrie Medford, C.N.
      International Standard Book Number: 0-9676419-6-9
      1. Nutrition 2. Health 3. Self Improvement I.Title

NOTE: This book is not intended to take the place of medical advice. Readers are advised to consult their doctor or other qualified healthcare professional regarding treatment of their medical conditions.

Printed in the United States of America

Second printing, 2007

(For ordering information, refer to the back pages of this book.)

The names of my clients have been changed. Any similarity to a real person is purely coincidental.

Contents

Foreword

In *Why Do I Feel So Lousy?* Lorrie Medford has done it, again. Lorrie has shown in all her previous books that she can take topics that are, in themselves, quite complicated and make them understandable, pleasant to read, and immediately useful. But, more importantly, Lorrie speaks from personal experience. She has been there, done that, and knows how to avoid "THAT" in the future!

This is an important book for YOU. As the world around us seems to be in constant turmoil with ever-increasing concerns for truly global problems, you might wonder what YOU can do to help. I would submit that the first, and perhaps the most important, thing you can do is to OBTAIN and MAINTAIN your personal health! When you are healthy, feeling good, and thinking clearly, then who knows what changes you might help bring about?

Those days when you just feel lousy are not the best for making decisions, relating to others, balancing your checkbook, or doing much of anything important. Lorrie's goal is to show you some simple, yet powerful, tools to help you take care of one of the most important organs of your body: Your LIVER. She clearly explains what this marvelous organ does and how important it is to YOU everyday. You may have heard your friends or someone else talk about doing a "detox" program, or "cleansing," or doing a "purification program" and wondered just what that is all about. Must I join a new fringe group and wear special clothing? Will my family still talk to me? You have the answers in your hands right now.

Supporting the body's effort to keep itself healthy and running efficiently is not difficult, but it will take some unlearning of wrong concepts and learning (or re-learning) some correct ones. Why should I eat Brussels sprouts? Do I have to eat cauliflower? What IS kale? Can I still have a cheeseburger? These and many other questions will be answered as you join Lorrie in her exploration of your liver and its relationship to your health.

I see the results of these principles in my practice every day. I have seen the results of practicing these principles in my own body. I used to weigh 120 pounds more than I do now, but that was years ago. I KNOW how hard it is to give up the "junk," but YOU can do it. You CAN make significant changes in your health NOW. The time to begin is NOW. You have the instruction manual in your hands. Open and read. Learn and do. Somebody out there needs YOU at your BEST—please let them have it!

Michael D. Dobbins, D. C.
Dobbins Affordable Chiropractic
Alameda, California

Acknowledgements

Many thanks to several of my clients who have given me permission to reprint their testimonies in this book.

I'm really grateful to Dr. Michael Dobbins who was gracious enough to re-read several versions of this book, (in the midst of an incredibly busy schedule!), to write the foreword to this book, and to allow me to interview him. Thanks for your commitment to teach nutrition in its many aspects around the country, all while you make us laugh!

Special thanks to Dr. Donna Smith, a practicing Certified Clinical Nutritionist, for her wonderful edit, feedback, and professional comments which brought further insight to the reader.

Many thanks to Charlie DuBois, Walter Scott, Hugh St. Onge, Tim Bahan, Joseph Antell, Randy DeWeerdt, Louis Trachtenberg, Vicki O'Brien, Jerry McFarland, Lewis Ruffner, Curt Hamilton, Glen Kikel, Donna Lannom, and Rick Toal for taking the time out of your busy schedules to read and encourage me in writing this book. Also, special thanks to Dr. Bruce Bond and Dr. Janet Lang for allowing me to quote you in this book.

I'm so grateful for my own staff, Carolyn Clark and Anne Spears who support both the the writing part and the client part of my practice. You are precious jewels! Many thanks, too, to Lori Oller, for her editing skills and great feedback. I'm also grateful to two of my clients, Mary Ferguson and Jim Wideman who were so gracious to share the results of their cleansing experience. I'm grateful for all of your comments, but I'm especially grateful for all of your questions which helped me clarify parts of this book.

I also thank Annie Gentil for her editorial comments and help with trademark and registration information. Many thanks also to both Ann Holden and Tammi Geiger for reading the manuscript and for your most helpful and encouraging comments. Finally, I thank the rest of the Standard Process staff involved in creating and educating us about their new Standard Process cleanse products.

Many thanks also to creative artist Tim Jurgensen for the book cover.

As I travel around the country and meet other teachers, nutritionists, and doctors, I'm so aware that there are hundreds or even thousands of people who understand nutrition at a level I could never begin to understand, especially the doctors I interviewed in this book. I always wonder why God didn't have them write these books! Each time I sit down, though, the books just come together in front of me! Clearly, it's something beyond myself. So finally, I thank God. Without God, I would not know, nor have, nor be anything. Without God, I would not know how to pursue life or my purpose for living.

Testimonies

Dear Lorrie,

"When I first started coming to you, I was very over weight, my cholesterol was sky high, and my blood pressure was also high. I was having trouble with cramps and pain in my side as well as dizziness. Immediately I started taking supplements, but what really made the big difference in my health was when I started doing a cleanse. Each time I would do a cleanse I would immediately feel better. It always jump started my weight loss, but more than that, I am pleased to announce that the cramps and side pain are gone, my blood pressure is normal and I'm off blood pressure medicine. My cholesterol is under 200 for the first time since I've been checking it. The dizziness is gone as well. I am a firm believer in cleansing now, in fact I am just finishing up one at the time of this writing. Thanks, Lorrie, for helping me to feel better and be healthier than I've been in years."

Jim W.

Dear Lorrie,

"As you know, I had a random rash for eight months. When it got to the legs, I had 2 doses of steroids. The doctor told me to take Allegra® and Benedryl®, which I didn't want to take because they didn't always help. When I did the cleanse that you recommended, it completely left. And I've lost 12 pounds. I sincerely thank you for your help."

Angela

Dear Lorrie,

"Since I've been coming to see you, my body is lighter and my mind is clearer. I wake up earlier. I can't remember ever feeling this good. I don't even need to take my allergy medications!"

Darlene

Dear Lorrie,

"I came to see you when I was diagnosed with Rheumatoid Arthritis. You recommended that I follow your detoxification program. After following the cleanse for two weeks, all of my knuckle pain left. My fasting blood sugars dropped to an average around 82 instead of 100. My blood pressure has come down and stayed normal without any drugs. For the last 10 months, anything strenuous has resulted in pain. In March I did two days of heavy shoveling and dirt moving for a new garden and had no knuckle pain at all."

David

Dear Lorrie,

"I've lost 10 pounds and feel great after following your program. I'm no longer constipated and I don't have headaches any more. My skin is clearing up as well. Thanks for all your help."

Paula

Dear Lorrie,

"My hot flashes are gone since I started the cleanse. And I've been able to lose the weight I gained over Christmas. I never knew that it would be this easy; I appreciate all of your help in learning how to cleanse my body and eat better, Lorrie."

Karen

Why Don't We Feel Well?

Something's wrong with us. In spite of all the doctors, and sophisticated medical equipment today, millions of Americans are sick and tired, or as I wrote in the title of my energy book, they are grumpy, dopey and sleepy!

Why do we spend billions of dollars annually on health and weight loss products and yet we still feel lousy?

Most people find that as they get older, things start to break down. Perhaps they gain weight or have high cholesterol levels for the first time in their lives. Or, they begin to have migraines, digestive problems, insomnia, or aches and pains. They may feel as though they are aging quicker. Isn't there anything they can do? Yes!

Despite medical breakthroughs, heart disease, cancer and diabetes are on the rise. The World Health Organization ranked the U.S. number one in healthcare spending, but the U.S. ranks thirty-seventh in overall quality of health. Japan is ranked number one in life expectancy even though their health care costs are 50% less than that of the U.S.

We spend more on medical care than any other nation in the world, but we're sicker than many of these nations. This book will show you how to invest in **true** health care.

What Could Be Wrong?

Marilyn, one of my clients, said, "Before I went to Lorrie, I suffered for years with a yeast infection that never cleared up, no matter what the doctor prescribed. After visiting Lorrie, the symptoms cleared up in 11 days! Through the years, she's also helped me eliminate symptoms of irritable bowel, migraines, psoriasis, bladder infections, daily nose bleeds, arthritis and anemia. I haven't had a cold or flu in five years! And best of all, I no longer struggle with sweet or chocolate cravings."

People come to my office with hundreds of symptoms of nutritional or hormonal imbalances, all of which can be helped with the natural solutions I'll present in this book. They include but are not limited to:

• High-blood pressure	• Gout
• Strokes	• Obesity
• Gallbladder disease	• Diabetes
• Heart attacks	• Sluggish liver
• Allergies	• Candida Albicans
• Osteoporosis	• Excessive stress
• Poor digestion and malabsorption	• Constipation
• Celiac Sprue disease	• Psoriasis
• Skin problems	• Insomnia
• Diverticulitis	• Toxic liver or bloodstream
• Crohn's disease	• Ulcers

People Need Help

I wrote this book for people who can't lose weight no matter what they try. Or for people who feel "lousy" or believe they have some type of health problem, but for some reason, their doctor can't find anything wrong. Or for the person who wants a natural solution for their poor digestion, chronic constipation and weight gain. Or for the person who is tired of taking allergy shots, blood-pressure medications, hormone replacement therapy, or diet pills, all of which have either produced:

1. No results.

2. Only temporary symptom relief.

3. Side effects of drugs that cause even more health problems.

The list could go on because nearly every person alive complains of some chronic condition that could be helped with amazingly simple changes in diet and lifestyle.

We're Supposed To Be Healthy!

Every part of our digestion and metabolism was designed to keep us active for a full, long life. Our bodies are incredibly designed with self-healing processes, provided we take care of them. If we're not healthy, somewhere along the way **we** have interfered with our body's normal process of healing.

And how do you explain those people who seem healthy, but aren't? Perhaps they exercised regularly, didn't drink alcohol, and didn't smoke. Yet one day they "mysteriously" got sick or even died of heart disease or cancer. How could this happen to such wonderful people? How could they be so easily caught in the web of disease? You'll see in this book, that waiting until we have physical symptoms before we think about good nutrition and following a healthy lifestyle is often too late. Learning about how to prevent disease is far better than trying to cure it!

How Nutrition Helps

A client named Elizabeth said, "I came to see Lorrie with a laundry list of complaints, all of which just occurred this year. I was tired, got sick frequently, had severe PMS symptoms, weight gain and pain in my muscles. I've been with Lorrie for six months and nearly every symptom is gone!"

Another client named Amy said, "I came to see Lorrie because of anemia and headaches. A friend told me about her and I thought maybe she could help. I was so excited! In the first month, I no longer had headaches, and my fatigue is gone. It's a shame we aren't taught how to take care of our bodies."

You Didn't Get an Owner's Manual

For centuries, clinical studies have proven that the better we eat, the healthier we are. But when were you taught about your body's natural healing processes? Much of the material presented in our educational system is outdated and it doesn't prepare us to live long and healthy lives.

Because of lack of education, we take better care of our cars than we do our bodies. You wouldn't, for example, put cheap fuel in your car. But few people realize the impact of foods on their health, or even know what "good" foods are.

You wouldn't let your car go a year without a tune-up or an oil change, yet most people go their entire lives without a tune-up for their bodies. You would never let your car battery run low, yet millions of Americans are fatigued almost to exhaustion. And you certainly wouldn't go for a year without washing your car. When was the last time you cleaned up on the inside? Probably never! It's worth the time it takes to check your own fuel, regenerate your batteries, get a tune-up and assist your body's natural internal cleansing process. Isn't your body worth more than your car?

More than 30 years ago, my father died of cancer. His death motivated me to spend the last 30 years studying the process of disease and how to **prevent** it. I've learned that good health is not an accident.

By the time you finish reading this book, you will understand what disease really is, and how to help your body get well, whether you want to lose weight, lower cholesterol or high-blood pressure, or gain more energy.

You'll see that we are not at the mercy of some heart disease or cancer gene, but that disease is the result of our interfering with our body's healing process. You'll see how sickness begins at the cell level, and it takes years before it might show up as symptoms. You'll also see how amazingly simple it really is to prevent, and possibly reverse, health problems with safe and effective, natural solutions.

14

Where Do You Need Help?

Throughout this book you'll see that it's more important to find and correct the **cause** than to just cover up **symptoms.**

I'll show you how to assist your body's **normal healing** processes. First, I'll walk you through a check-up to determine your current health profile. Then I'll show you how to do a tune-up which can take years off your age, help you feel great, lose weight, and even begin the process of reversing disease.

I'll also be presenting a clinical program I've used with thousands of clients. I'll refer you to "natural" health professionals. These include: Naturopathic Doctors (N.D.), Clinical Nutritionists (C.N.), Certified Clinical Nutritionists (C.C.N.), and doctors (D.C., M.D., D.D., D.O., D.D.S., Ph.D.) who have studied Clinical Nutrition (see Appendix.)

No matter who you are, the ideas and suggestions in this book will help you to get healthy. You don't have to feel lousy! Getting your health back is more than just a health issue; it's a life issue!

Below is a list of the parts of this book. You can read it all the way through, or just read the chapters that interest you. I've included lots of charts with bullets so you can get through the chapters quickly.

• *Part One looks at toxins, the symptoms of toxicity inside and outside of us and their link to disease and feeling lousy.*

• *Part Two contains your check-up. You'll find several tests to determine your current health profile.*

• *Part Three begins your tune-up, starting with your stomach, liver and elimination as related to disease and feeling lousy.*

• *Part Four presents dozens of benefits for changing your diet using specific foods.*

• *Part Five gives you an incredible solution to healing. You'll be amazed at the hundreds of "diseases" helped through internal cleansing.*

I've also included Endnotes and an Index for those who like to do additional research. Let's get started on your journey to vitality.

PART ONE

Why Do We Feel Lousy?

Chapter One

Me, Toxic?

It seems everyone is chasing after the magic diet or pill that will help them increase their energy, lose weight and stop aging. And even after taking the latest vitamin pills and wrinkle creams, we still seem to be more tired and toxic!

A client named Amy, had fatigue and headaches for years until she started my nutritional program. On a follow-up appointment, she said, "We are so used to having a complaint and going to our doctor. He puts us on a drug for the rest of our lives. We don't complain because the pain is gone. But we never really fixed the problem; and no one tells us that the drugs the doctor gave us could be toxic, hard for our liver to eliminate, and eventually cause more problems."

In this chapter I'll show you common symptoms of toxicity, what toxins are, where they are, and how they make us feel lousy! Let's start with common symptoms of toxicity.

Common Symptoms of Toxicity

- Fatigue
- Weight gain and/or cellulite
- Dark circles under eyes
- PMS
- Pale skin
- Metallic taste in mouth
- Difficulty sleeping
- Mentally dull
- Hypoglycemia
- Allergies
- Skin conditions
- Diarrhea
- High-blood pressure
- Low libido
- Yellowing or discoloration of whites of the eyes

- Food cravings
- Indigestion or reflux
- Puffiness under the eyes
- Frequent headaches
- Coated tongue
- Gas and bloating
- Joint pain
- Dry skin
- Fibromyalgia
- High cholesterol
- Poor digestion
- Fluid retention
- Irregular periods
- Constipation

Notice fatigue and weight gain are listed at the top. Your body has to be healthy to properly burn fat or have energy. Weight gain, and any other symptoms you may have accepted as normal can also be reduced or eliminated through the program I'll show you in this book. But first, what is a toxin?

What Is a Toxin?

A toxin is either a foreign substance we take into our body that harms it and hinders it from healing (such as a chemical) or one that our body creates as a by-product of metabolism (waste). Unfortunately, one of the most common ways to become toxic is through our American diet!

Of course there is no magic pill. But the way to increase energy, lose weight and slow the aging process is to support your body's natural ability to eliminate toxins.

Toxins in Our Food Supply

The fast-food American diet of high-fat, sugar, and salt does not give our bodies enough nutrients to maintain proper health and hinders our normal internal cleansing abilities.

Recently, a male client came to see me complaining of severe fatigue. I explained to Jerone that fatigue can occur because of two reasons: Vitamin deficiencies and/or toxicity. We consider third-world people malnourished, yet even overweight Americans can be starving for good nutrition.

The foods that cause vitamin deficiencies are the same ones that are toxic and make us tired. The four most common substances in the average American diet listed below could be called the "Four Food Groups!" (This is a short list. For more complete information, see my books listed at the end of this book.)

1. Refined white sugar

Americans eat approximately 200 pounds of sugar per person, per year. We were designed to handle between 10-25 pounds. Do you know what happens to the excess?

Consuming high amounts of sugar is a risk factor for heart disease. In an article in his *Medical Letter,* Dr. John R. Lee explains how "the cholesterol scam" has been blamed for heart disease for years. His advice is to reduce the American addiction to sugar and refined carbohydrates, which are the real culprits in causing low HDL, cholesterol and oxidized LDL cholesterol.[1] Additionally, excess sugar is linked to diabetes and many other diseases.

Eating sugar causes deficiencies of the B complex, and minerals such as zinc, all vital for a healthy immune system. Having one serving of sugar (3-6 teaspoons) depresses our immune system for the next 6-8 hours.

Finally, consuming excess amounts of sugar has a detrimental affect on the endocrine system and the liver, causing the same kind of liver damage as alcohol could.   (I highly recommend Nancy Appleton's book, *Lick the Sugar Habit,* as well my energy book, *Why Am I So Grumpy, Dopey and Sleepy?*, and weight-loss book, *Why Can't I Lose Weight?)*

It's not always easy for people to give up substances they like, though. When my mother read my book about sugar and the problems it causes, she gave up reading!

2. Refined white flour

Refined white flour originally came from whole grains.   In the process of making white flour, nearly all the vitamins and minerals are eliminated in the refining process, including 98% of vitamin E and 70-80% of the B vitamins, including folic acid. These are nutrients that protect our heart from damage. Dr. Royal Lee, a genius and pioneer in clinical nutrition, considered consuming white flour one of the leading causes of heart disease.[2]

The high heat and pressure used in the processing of puffed grains makes the grains toxic. In his book, *Fighting the Food Giants,* Paul Stitt reported an experiment where rats were fed whole wheat or puffed wheat. The rats who ate the whole wheat lived more than a year, while the rats that ate the puffed wheat died within two weeks.[3]

Additionally, white flour contributes to toxicity because the precious fiber is eliminated during the processing. As you'll see later in this book, fiber is vital for proper bowel function and the removal of toxins.

3. Processed fats and oils

For years, we thought that to lose weight and have low cholesterol, we needed to follow a low-fat diet. Today, we know that we desperately need "good" essential fats and oils for good health and weight management. What we need to eliminate are the processed fats. As with the sugar and flour examples, the processing of the fats makes them toxic, too.

Fried foods are toxic foods. When oils are heated above 300 degrees Fahrenheit, the natural cis-fatty acid molecules are changed into a toxic category of fats called, "trans fats." These fats have been implicated in a number of diseases, including heart disease and breast cancer.

Fats that are hydrogenated, such as oils used in the making of margarine are also considered trans fats. (An excellent book about fats and oils is *Fats That Heal, Fats that Kill* by Udo Erasmus.)

4. Caffeine (coffee, soda, chocolate or tea)

According to author Dr. Linda Berry, in her book, *Internal Cleansing,* the caffeine in your coffee belongs in the same alkaloid group of chemicals as morphine and cocaine, and caffeine users have a 100% greater than average risk of a heart attack.[4]

Coffee is toxic because growers use heavy amounts of pesticides on coffee crops, and the roasting process turns the oils in coffee into trans fats.[5] This can cause congestion of the liver, and also hinder fat loss.

I've also discovered that it's hard to lose weight drinking soda, including the "diet" types. Additionally, did you know that there is more sugar in a can of soda than in a bag of cotton candy?

Toxins in Our Environment

We're surrounded with toxins! We drink them, eat them and breathe them into our body. Our body produces toxins through its normal metabolic processes. Our crops are sprayed with fungicides and pesticides. Chemicals are sprayed on coffee beans.

Beef and chicken are given growth hormones to increase their weight, and dairy cows are injected with hormones to increase their milk production. All of these hormones are stored in the animal's tissues. When we later eat these animals, we also ingest these hormones. These growth hormones can adversely affect both male and female hormone balance. (An example is PMS, or as we affectionately call it, Punish My Spouse!) Additionally, it's also common to give beef cattle antibiotics, which again, our bodies ingest.

When was the last time you took an antibiotic? People take them frequently, but did you know that their use has set up a condition of toxicity that our bodies were not designed to handle? What occurs from the use of antibiotics is that our natural healthy flora, or bacteria in the colon, that help us defend against pathogenic germs begins to decrease. This then leads to an overgrowth of germs that, in turn, secrete by-products which are also toxic to our system.

You've probably heard that our homes are also subject to many toxic chemicals. It's no wonder you might sneeze a lot after moving into a new home! For example, cleaning products, synthetic carpets, upholstery and drapes all contain toxic vapors. The beautiful lawns that most Americans are so proud of contain 50% of the pesticides used in the U.S.

The 1989 Kellogg Report stated that 1,000 newly synthesized compounds are introduced each year. That amounts to three new chemicals a day. The current number of known xenobiotics (foreign chemicals) now totals around 100,000 and includes drugs, pesticides, industrial chemicals, food additives and environmental pollutants. Unfortunately, the Environmental Protection Agency (EPA) hasn't even begun to test these chemicals for safety. Uh-oh!

Here's a short list of other common toxins that people expect their body to handle, yet they really can't! So they feel —you guessed it! Lousy!

- Secondhand smoke
- Cleaning materials
- Pesticides and herbicides
- Lead or mercury
- Silicone breast implants
- Industrial pollutants
- Smoking
- Indoor pollutants (such as from carpets)
- Car exhaust
- Some cosmetics
- Air pollution
- Prescription drugs
- Radiation
- Steroids

What About Our Foods?

Prior to World War II, farmers used crop rotation to control pests. Authors of the well-researched book, *Is our Food Safe?*, Warren Leon and Caroline Smith DeWaal write that pesticides have dramatically increased the amount of food grown without increasing the amount of farmland required. Today, farmers are the heaviest users of pesticides. **These authors point out that we have no way of knowing what and how much of a pesticide is in our food.** Unfortunately, the effects of toxic chemicals in foods may not be evident for years after chemicals have been ingested. Additionally, they report that in 1987, the EPA estimated that pesticide residues on food might cause cancer in as many as 6,000 people annually in the United States![6]

I found it interesting that 90% of herbicide applications are applied to just four crops: Corn, soybeans, cotton and wheat.[7] Besides the refining process, this may explain why these foods seem to cause the most allergies in people.

Finally, they explain the importance of having stricter standards for our drinking water. They report that the Center for Disease Control and Prevention (CDC) estimates about 940,000 Americans get sick and 900 die each year from water-borne microbial illnesses caused by drinking water.[8]

How Do Toxins Make Us Sick?

Our bodies do the best they can, but there is a limit to how much "good" health you can experience in the process. When we continue, year after year, to demand that our body handle an overload of toxins that it was not designed to handle, sooner or later, symptoms of disease appear.

Did you ever wonder what happens to these chemicals and toxins in our body if they are not processed and eliminated?

They find their way into the blood and are then stored in the tissues of the body. They overload the eliminative organs, especially the liver, and **as a result, most Americans are fatigued and/or overweight and feel just plain lousy!**

Clinical research shows us that a person's risk of cancer is related to their level of nutrition and their body's ability to process toxins. The body's inability to handle toxins may be a determining factor in most diseases. The better your body can eliminate toxins, the more likely you'll be healthy.

Toxins Weaken our Immune System

When I was young I was taught that germs caused disease. I finally realized that my symptoms were not due to some bad germs, (for example, bacteria or fungus) but rather, a weak body that created the environment for germs and bacteria to eat and thrive.

The fast foods we commonly eat, most of which contain sugar, not only give germs something to eat, but serve these germs a five-course meal! That's another reason why eating sugar makes you sicker; it feeds the bad guys!

Wouldn't it be helpful if we felt the effect of toxins immediately? Of course, we usually have little idea of their presence.

But, sooner or later, symptoms of toxicity will show up. They can cause damage long before you see or experience symptoms. Remember, they are attacking your body at the cell level and you may not feel it until the cellular damage progresses to tissue degeneration or organ/gland dysfunction. In other words, you start to get aches and pains!

According to author and nutritionist Dr. Patrick Quillin, toxins lower immune function and damage DNA.[9]

Unseen DNA changes may even affect your offspring and many years later, their offspring. This can explain how a child can be born with a serious disease, such as cancer.

How Toxins Affect Us

Toxins, from chemicals to pesticides to additives, can affect every part of our body. I've summarized a list of the ways that toxins can hurt our system from the *Seven Day Detox Miracle* by Peter Bennett.[10]

Toxins can affect:

• The digestive system causing gas, bloating, indigestion and constipation or diarrhea.

• The musculoskeletal system causing pain, numbness or tingling and fatigue.

• The immune system causing a weakened system, frequent colds, or allergies, autoimmune diseases, arthritis, neurological diseases, heart diseases and cancer.

• The central nervous system causing poor memory or lack of concentration (including stress and anxiety).

• The skin by causing itching, hives, or psoriasis.

What About Your Toxic Load?

You might be wondering how you would know if you are toxic? Really, your body is giving you answers all the time! Here are questions I commonly ask my clients to get an idea of their toxic load.

Check the following if they apply to you:

1. Do you drink tap water?
2. Do you eat fast foods frequently?
3. Do you drink coffee regularly?
4. Do you use artificial sweeteners regularly?
5. Do you often drink beer or wine or other alcoholic drinks?
6. Do you drink soda or diet soft drinks?
7. Do you frequently buy foods that contain chemical preservatives or other additives (that you can't pronounce)?
8. Do you commonly eat foods such as candy, cake and ice cream?
9. Do you eat French fries regularly?
10. Do you eat potato chips or corn chips regularly?
11. Do you eat commercial meat and chicken instead of organic meats and chicken?
12. Do you eat commercial fruits and vegetables instead of organic fruits and vegetables?

If the majority of your answers are yes, then it is likely that your diet significantly increases your toxic load.

Obviously, we will continue to be exposed to environmental toxins. So what can we do about it?

Of course, we can take steps to change our diets and to eat healthier foods. You'll learn more about this later in this book.

Additionally, we need to cleanse our bodies from the inside out! You know, kind of giving your internal organs and glands a nice shower. You can do this by eating common, healthy foods that assist your body to cleanse, and taking cleansing nutritional supplements. You don't have to grow a beard, or join a special cult! This type of nutritional therapy is called detoxification, or "internal" cleansing.

The idea of internal cleansing has been around for centuries and it's also well documented. In Europe, for example, detoxification or internal cleansing is considered a medical therapy and is used in mainstream medical doctors' offices and spas.

Your body needs very specific nutrients in order to eliminate these toxins. In a clinical setting, this type of therapy could be called a "detoxification" program. Since the word "detox" is often involved in detoxifying people from drugs and alcohol, for the purpose of simplicity, in this book I refer to it as an "internal cleanse."

There are many good cleansing (detoxifying) programs available. Of course, I'm going to write about the eating plan and nutritional therapy that I've used personally and professionally with hundreds of clients in my practice. Chapter 7 will have details on this program.

But before we get to the cleansing part, let's take a look at the organs of digestion and cleansing along the way.

Let's now go to your nutritional check-up in part 2.

PART TWO

What About You?

Chapter Two

Do You Need a Check-Up?

Like most people, I grew up eating what my family ate. My twin worked at a donut factory when we were in college. I remember meeting her at 5:00 a.m. so we could both eat as many jelly-filled donuts as we could pack in. Ummm! It never occurred to me that's why I had acne, a weight problem, or I had to take a nap several times that day! We both liked donuts, and we didn't think about what they were doing to us internally. (They weren't even Krispy Kreme!®)

Watching our father die of cancer was a wake-up call for us. We learned that nutritional deficiencies could, and did, cause physical imbalances that eventually caused disease. I'll never forget our response to this knowledge: Why weren't we told before now? My older sister influenced my twin sister and I to change our diets, and as a result, we really felt better. It was the beginning of our lifelong passion for health.

Cause and Effect Nutrition

The food that we eat has an effect on our cells. It either nourishes them or damages them. If we are well nourished, we are healthy, and if we aren't nourished, then we become sick or begin the aging and degeneration process.

Consider that each year we consume about four pounds of chemical preservatives and additives. Did you ever wonder what happens to all of these chemicals? Did you think, like I did, that our body just processes everything perfectly? Most people never consider what happens if we can't break down and eliminate these chemicals.

I asked Dr. Bruce Bond, a chiropractor who teaches nutrition, what specifically happens to these chemicals. He says, "The long-term ingestion of chemicals and toxins leads to what we label 'disease.'" Dr. Bond says that our bodies only have three options when it comes to these chemicals and toxins:[11]

1. Bury them in body fat
2. Deposit them in tissues
3. Eliminate them.

As you might think, the first two options aren't good ones. Imagine what would happen if you never changed the oil in your car. I'm not very mechanically minded, but even I know that's not good!

So many chronic problems that people consider to be a natural part of aging are really the result of a build-up of chemicals and toxins that our body was designed to break down and eliminate, but it can't for some reason.

Your Body is Amazing

Our bodies have a type of oil filter too! It's your liver. Every few minutes your blood circulates through the liver. The liver uses several processes to break down various chemicals and toxins so your body can eliminate them. **Our body is designed to constantly heal itself.** It accomplishes this through various internal "cleansing" processes which depend on simple foods such as broccoli. Unfortunately, these are the foods no one wants to eat! What happens if we don't eat these foods? It becomes continually harder for the liver to break down the chemicals and cleanse the blood.

Can We Handle it?

In my weight-loss book, I quoted nutritionist, Dr. Lindsey Duncan, who said, "Under ideal circumstances, the body is well equipped to neutralize and dispose of toxins through the liver, spleen and eliminative channels (i.e., bowel, kidneys, lungs, skin and lymphatic system). But in modern day society there are no ideal circumstances."[12] Duncan further says that most of us have been raised on foods, such as fast foods, that interfere with the digestive and eliminative process.

Because people eat foods all day long that contain chemical preservatives or additives, our bodies are overburdened and cannot ideally do the job they were designed to do.

(Did you know why it's called "fast" food? Because it's designed to be eaten fast; otherwise, you might be able to taste it!)

So what does all this mean? Through my research and my practice, I've identified four stages of disease.

1. Poor digestion
2. A sluggish liver
3. Poor elimination
4. A weakened immune system

Stage One: Poor Digestion

Food that is not broken down properly doesn't just cause a stomachache; it causes future health problems! Undigested food putrefies and ferments in the stomach and is turned into a toxic substance which later passes from the blood into the tissues. And all without you even knowing about it!

From working with thousands of clients, I've discovered that dozens of health and energy problems stem from poor digestion. Here's a short list:

Mental fatigue, lack of concentration, memory loss, insomnia, nightmares, heartburn, gas, nausea, burping, abdominal pain, diarrhea, constipation, all types of allergies, gallstones, chronic indigestion, obesity, adult-onset diabetes, premature aging, arthritis, lowered immunity, cardiovascular disease, and poor hormone production.

Your First Check-Up

I'm reprinting three simple tests for you from my first book, *Why Can't I Lose Weight?*[13] which will quickly help you understand how strong your digestion currently is.

Check the following if it applies to you:

1. Do you ever burp after meals?
2. Do you get stomachaches?
3. Do you overeat regularly?
4. Do you need to take an antacid after every meal?
5. Do you have indigestion regularly?
6. Do you often have heartburn or reflux?
7. Do you have gas or bloating after meals?
8. Do you have constipation or diarrhea?
9. Do you experience fatigue after eating?
10. Do you suffer from allergies?
11. Do you have dark circles under your eyes?
12. Do you have greasy or poorly-formed stools?

If you answered yes to even one of these symptoms, you may have trouble with your stomach and digestion. (See chapter 3.)

Stage Two: A Sluggish Liver

The second part of your check-up is your liver. In her most fascinating book, *The Healthy Liver and Bowel Book,* (great bathroom reading!) Australian Doctor Sandra Cabot lists the many, many symptoms associated with liver dysfunction. They include:[14]

• **Abnormal metabolism of fats** including cellulite, weight gain, fat around the middle, pot belly, high cholesterol and triglycerides.

• **Digestive problems,** including reflux, gallstones, nausea, irritable bowel and pain in the liver.

• **Blood sugar problems,** including cravings for sugar.

• **Nervous system problems,** including depression, mood swings and foggy brain.

• **Immune dysfunction,** including allergies, skin rashes, Chronic Fatigue Syndrome, and Fibromyalgia.

• **Hormonal imbalance,** including menopausal symptoms and PMS.

Wow! Who would have ever thought that a sluggish liver was related to so many symptoms!

Check the following if it applies to you:
1. Do you have a hormonal imbalance (both men and women)?
2. Do you suffer from moodiness, irritability, and confusion?
3. Do you have PMS (irregular menstrual cycle, cramps, or breast tenderness)?
4. Do you often feel bloated?
5. Do you have high cholesterol?
6. Do you have eye problems?
7. Do you have a coated tongue?
8. Do you have bad breath?
9. Do you have problems with low-blood sugar?
10. Do you get chilled after a meal?
11. Do you have frequent headaches?
12. Do you have an eating disorder?
13. Do you have skin diseases and problems (including pigment or deposits on the back of the hands)?
14. Do you have frequent nausea?
15. Do you have frequent allergies?
16. Do you have constipation and/or diarrhea?

If you answered yes to one or more of the questions in this section, your liver needs help. (See chapter 4.)

Stage Three: Poor Elimination

The third part of your check-up is your colon. It's not just what we eat, but it's what we absorb, assimilate and eliminate that matters. (That's a mouthful!) Our 26 feet of digestive tract can keep us young and full of energy, or lead us to disease and premature death.

Unfortunately, the colon lining gradually becomes damaged when we continually eat such things as ice cream, candy, sweets, fried and fast foods. We feel it happening because later we become tired, experience gas, bloating, brain fog, low-blood sugar, headaches and constipation! Trapped toxins and waste pollute our bloodstream. This leads to digestive problems and eventually disease when we don't internally cleanse the colon.

Check the following if it applies to you:

1. Do you suffer from chronic constipation, diarrhea or both?
2. Do you have a bloated, distended, tender or rigid abdomen?
3. Do you have regular gas and flatulence?
4. Do you suffer from colitis?
5. Do you have poor circulation?
6. Are you overweight?
7. Do you have chronic lower-back pain?
8. Do you have bad breath?
9. Do you have bad body odor (feet, hands, under arms)?
10. Do you have frequent headaches?
11. Do you have a poor appetite or abnormal cravings for food?
12. Do you have skin problems or acne?

If you answered yes to one or more of these symptoms, you need to internally cleanse your colon. (See chapter 5.)

Stage Four: Weakened Immune System

At this stage, toxins are rampant and the elimination system is so impaired that now the symptoms of pain, swelling and inflammation occur. As you'll see later in this book, chronic pain can be related to a body that can't handle all the toxins!

The immune system is now weakened and this eventually leads to further degeneration and disease. If your body can't eliminate waste, toxins can accumulate in your body as cysts, polyps or tumors. That will get your attention!

Disease doesn't necessarily happen in a month, or a year. Disease comes from toxic accumulation over years, and years and years. The disease process can even start in children. I've heard that autopsies performed on teens show early stages of heart disease. Put simply, we have waited too long for our check-up and we desperately need a tune-up!

Check the following if it applies to you:

1. Do you have brain fog?
2. Do you have watery, itchy eyes?
3. Do you have aches or pains in your joints?
4. Do you have a chronic cough or sinus problems?
5. Do you have shortness of breath or asthma?
6. Do you have allergies?
7. Do you have constipation or diarrhea?
8. Do you experience hot flashes or an overheating of the body?
9. Do you feel groggy upon awakening?
10. Do you frequently have headaches?
11. Do you have root canals or mercury amalgam fillings?
12. Do you have bags or circles under your eyes?
13. Do you frequently feel depressed or experience low energy levels?
14. Do you suffer from frequent infections or chemical sensitivities?

If you answered yes to one or more of these questions, you'll want to help strengthen your immune system with the internal cleansing program in this book.

Most of us live without ever considering these stages of degeneration. Most of us don't even know why we get a stomachache or any other pain for that matter!

Your internal parts are so important! But no one ever tells us how to take care of them! No wonder we can feel so lousy.

So let's move on to part 3 where you will learn more about your stomach, liver and colon and how they support your body's own healing and cleansing process.

PART THREE

How To Get Beyond Indigestion

Chapter Three

Should You Really Eat Everything?

I find it interesting that we think so many symptoms of poor digestion are "normal." These symptoms include heartburn, gas, bloating, ulcers and even reflux. It seems like everyone has them, and if they don't have them now, they are just expecting them! In fact, it's so common now to take a drug for an upset stomach, these symptoms are often seen as Tums®, Zantac® or Pepsid® deficiencies!

Drugs enable us to literally eat "anything" we want. In fact, there are now drugs we can take ahead of time just to insure we won't have stomach symptoms later. We are not taught to wonder what happens when we eat food, or how to avoid the foods that give us stomachaches. We just imagine that our body takes care of everything, because nothing bad happens to us immediately.

Our bodies are amazingly resilient! People can be symptom free in spite of their diet, not because of it. As you'll see in this book, the common American way of eating does more damage than good. The first place to consider, when you feel lousy for any reason, is your stomach.

In this chapter, I'll discuss common problems including stomachache, heartburn, gas, bloating, ulcers, reflux and food allergies, all of which affect your health. You're only as healthy as your digestion!

Oh, My Stomach Hurts!

Did it ever occur to you that having a stomachache is a natural response to something that you have eaten recently? Instead of taking a drug to get rid of the symptom, we should instead wonder what in the world we did to cause the problem.

Nearly everyone has experienced a stomachache. Perhaps it only happens when you eat at a Mexican restaurant, or after eating a rich dessert. We tend to ignore occasional pain, and we only take pain seriously when we have continual problems. But did you know that stomachaches are a signal that you are damaging your digestive tract? Rather than just take away the pain, we need to heal the digestive tract, and eliminate the source of the problem; for example, those foods that hurt the delicate lining of the stomach.

Factors That Cause Digestive Problems

• Eating fried foods	• Eating too fast
• Overusing antacids	• Not chewing well
• Eating too many fatty foods	• Overeating
• Not getting enough fiber	• Drinking alcohol
• Overeating red meat	• Smoking
• Drinking too much caffeine	• Eating artificial foods
• Eating white sugar	• Stress
• Eating refined carbohydrates	• Drinking soda

So What's An Enzyme?

Enzymes are a type of protein that help to digest, absorb, transport, metabolize, and eliminate waste. One of the most important jobs of enzymes is to digest our food, making it so small that it can pass through the minute openings of the intestines into the bloodstream.

The foods in the list above hinder our natural enzyme production. Enzymes are so vital that thousands of my clients have eliminated digestive problems by simply taking a digestive enzyme supplement.

How Enzymes Help

• They aid digestion	• They boost your energy
• They boost metabolism	• They help detoxify
• They help slow aging	• They help in weight loss
• They aid in a faster response to injury	

We are born with a certain number of enzymes or an "enzyme bank." Like your bank account, you make withdrawals every time you eat processed foods, sugar, white flour, fried foods or drink alcohol. However, once you run out, you need to replenish the account.

Enzymes are heat sensitive, so cooking foods over 118°F. destroys these vital enzymes. This includes cooking, baking, frying, and microwaving, or the American way of eating!

Most Americans eat mostly cooked foods and I've read that the average American spends as little as $2 a week on fresh produce. You would hope cooking improves the nutritional value of food! Unfortunately, it destroys or makes unavailable 85% of the original nutrients.

Many of my clients tell me that they don't have time to buy, eat or prepare vegetables. They are good candidates for enzyme supplementation! Read below to see if you are.

You Need Enzyme Supplements If You...

- Do not eat raw fruits & vegetables
- Have bowel or digestive problems
- Eat only cooked and processed foods
- Eat white sugar frequently
- Are a diabetic
- Are overweight
- Are under stress
- Overeat regularly
- Drink coffee or alcohol
- Smoke

I use enzymes made by a company called Standard Process®. (These are only sold through health professionals, so you will have to contact the health professional who sold you this book, or call the 1-800 number listed in the Appendix of this book to find someone to purchase them from.)

Hydrochloric Acid (HCl)

In addition to enzymes, your stomach also makes hydrochloric acid, or HCl, for breaking down protein. Americans start to have deficiencies of HCl at an average age of 35 to 45. This condition is known as hypochlorhydria, and it affects half of the people over age 50. Lack of HCl leads to many problems such as: Constipation, flatulence, and cramps.

Clinical Nutritionist Dr. Donna Smith says that if you were a bottle fed baby, you lose HCl sooner than if you were a breast fed baby. Even children can show a deficiency of this important nutrient when they cry with colic and cramps!

Symptoms of HCl Deficiency

- Bad breath
- Feeling full after eating
- Constipation
- Belching or nausea
- Weak, cracked, fingernails
- Skin problems such as eczema
- Bloating and gas
- Cramping
- Passage of undigested food
- Coated tongue
- Chronic yeast infections

Here are additional ways that HCl helps keep us healthy.

HCl Helps

- Maintain youthful vibrant body
- Regulate calcium metabolism
- Regulate menstruation for women
- Improve digestion and assimilation
- Fight germs and bacteria
- Maintain healthy skin
- Normalize the urine

Is Heartburn Your Problem?

If you watch any television at all, you'll think that if you have acid indigestion, or heartburn, that you have too much acid. Americans spend two billion dollars a year on antacids! Full-page advertisements for people with heartburn report that some two hundred and thirty-seven million prescriptions have been written for Tagamet®.[15] Antacids are called the "most prescribed medication of its kind" boasting of 550 million consumers. That adds up to an incredible number of people with what we call heartburn or sour stomachs!

But do they really have too much acid? Many of the clients I have seen actually don't produce enough acid! Therefore, this "acid indigestion" may be caused by not enough HCl. Here's what really happens.

Our stomach begins the process of digesting food with both digestive enzymes and HCl. As we age, our bodies produce less and less HCl. Without this **beneficial** acid, however, food stays in the stomach too long. Eventually, the food begins to ferment, **producing an extremely dangerous, toxic acid.** When people complain of an acid stomach, this is the acid that they are referring to, not the good HCl that we were born with.

What About Reflux?

Most people that I see who have an acidic stomach, also have what is commonly called "reflux." Often they are also either knowingly or unknowingly constipated! Doctors have named this "acid reflux disease" as if it just mysteriously appeared out of no where. No, it begins with the lack of HCl, and it then becomes a stomach, liver and colon problem.

Here's how it works. HCl in the stomach tells the small intestine to begin digestion. When the acid is low, the signal is weak. The stomach has to eliminate its contents, but instead of going down to the small intestine, the food goes back up the esophagus! Unfortunately, the esophagus lining isn't protected with a mucous layer like the stomach is. So the esophagus can become inflamed and you feel pain when this happens.

Another function of HCl is to send a signal to the liver to produce bile, which sends a signal to the colon to begin peristalsis, or the emptying of the bowel.

Since most people don't know how their body really works, and they are taught to stop the symptom instead of getting to the cause, they watch an ad on TV, and buy an antacid or worse, acid-blocking medications. Their symptoms stop. They feel fine. Problem solved. Or is it? What really happened here?

These drugs alleviate symptoms by neutralizing or blocking the body's production of stomach acid. I said earlier that not having enough HCl was linked to the passage of undigested food! So now, partially digested food is forced through the digestive tract. This is not how we were designed. **We are bypassing an important mechanism that**

39

was designed to keep us well! Let's look at the problems associated with these acid blockers.

Earlier I explained that we desperately need a proper supply of HCl. These drugs deal with the **symptoms**, but their action **stops digestion and absorption**. According to Dr. Janet Lang, a practicing chiropractor who teaches nutrition to doctors around the country, **"The consequence of the use of acid-blockers is dire and extreme, yet it is completely ignored by conventional medicine."** She lists five serious results of these drugs:[16]

1. **Malnutrition**. Proteins and most minerals can't be digested without a strong acid medium. Consequently, people begin to feed off their own protein (muscle and organs) and mineral (bone density) reserves. Additionally, pancreas and bile function are inhibited, causing malabsorption of all nutrients and fats.

2. **Toxicity**. When food isn't digested properly, it putrefies, and ferments. This results in toxicity, gas, bloating, diarrhea or constipation.

3. **Hypochlorhydria**. She says **any and all** disease processes are related to hypochlorhydria (lack of HCl).

4. **Parasites**. Without proper stomach function, people are susceptible to any type of food- or water-borne parasite.

5. **Degeneration of Gastric Mucosa**. A result of prolonged use of acid-stoppers is degeneration of the gastric mucosa (natural lining of the GI tract). This can cause debilitating fatigue, severe stomach pains and chronic diarrhea.

Dr. Lang says that no medical protocol can heal this situation. The goal is to assist normal digestion, and heal the gastric mucosa which can be done under the care of your natural health professional, such as the one who provided this book for you or who recommends Standard Process® supplements.

Dr. Lang says that until you stop using the acid-stopping medication (with your doctor's assistance), you won't get better. You will become more nutritionally deficient and your symptoms will only become worse. Read on for more information about HCl.

HCl Compared to Antacids

Let's compare HCl to most antacids.

HCl helps your body break down minerals such as calcium, magnesium and potassium. It also helps break down B12 and iron. Calcium deficiency, and B12 and iron deficiency anemias are often caused by lack of HCl. (I routinely recommend Zypan® by Standard Process® for these conditions.)

Antacids deal with the symptoms of poor digestion, however, they don't **assist** in digestion. So the nutrients from your foods, which depend on HCl, are poorly absorbed.

HCl is also required to break down protein. If you don't have enough HCl, undigested particles of protein pass through the digestive tract. This causes, at least, protein deficiency and at worse, could be the beginning of allergies.

Antacids don't contain HCl, so all digestion is compromised.

HCl destroys harmful bacteria and parasites.

Antacids are a cause of malabsorption and yeast overgrowth.

So the average person, not knowing any difference, buys an antacid such as Tums®. But Tums, or any antacid, is not the answer to the problem because it never gets to the root cause: Lack of HCl. Unfortunately, commercial antacids in wafers, powders, or bicarbonate of soda actually decrease the supply of HCl. This always adds to digestive trouble!

By the way, according to experts, Tums are a poorly absorbed source of calcium which provides a false sense of security that calcium needs are met. Dr. Michael Murray, author of *The Encyclopedia of Natural Medicine,* says that popular calcium carbonate antacids, such as Tums may actually **cause** kidney stones. He also reports that sodium bicarbonate antacids, such as Rolaids® also have side effects which can interfere with kidney and heart function. Aluminum magnesium compounds, such as Mylanta®, may cause phosphorus and calcium imbalances, and possible aluminum toxicity or accumulation of aluminum in the brain.[17]

Antacids can have serious side effects. In an article in *Health Counselor,* Dr. Michael Murray reports that Tagamet® and Zantac® are associated with digestive disturbances, nutritional imbalances, liver dysfunction, disruption of bone metabolism, and breast development in men.[18]

Secretion of HCl is the key to digestion of carbohydrates, proteins and fats. Additionally, HCl helps signal the release of bile which is made by the liver. So lack of HCl may cause an insufficient bile production which is vital for the digestion of fats and fat-soluble vitamins. This explains why just taking an enzyme with proper HCl can help the digestion of fats and consequently, weight loss.

Finally, HCl is also the spark that ignites the action of your intestines, which is a muscular motion called peristalsis. Like I tell my clients, constipation begins in the stomach when people don't have enough HCl!

Food Allergies

What happens when food that was supposed to be properly digested doesn't have the enzymes and HCl? Remember, most people don't know anything about how their stomach is supposed to work. We know where our stomach is, however, when it hurts!

Your body tries to "handle" food whether it has all of the proper digestive help or not. If foods are not broken down, they enter the bloodstream and are then recognized by the body as a "foreign invader" that it tries to eliminate. An example of this process could be sinus problems or when the body begins to attack itself as in autoimmune conditions, which is a highly toxic condition. All of these began because of poor digestion.

What Can You Do?

Make sure you have enough HCl in your stomach. A good way to determine if you are deficient in HCl is to take some apple cider vinegar or an enzyme with HCl (such as Zypan® by Standard Process®, manufacturer of whole-food supplements since 1929.) and see how it makes you feel. What if after taking Zypan® or apple cider vinegar, you feel worse?

Vicki O'Brien, a friend and researcher involved with whole-food supplementation, adds additional insight to this situation:

"More than 90% of people are not producing enough acid. If Zypan® or apple cider vinegar increases their discomfort then this is a good indication of the presence of a stomach ulcer. A person producing too much HCl is very rare. Instead, what is happening is that a person has too much acid from the acid produced by his rotting food, leading to stomach ulcers."

Vicki also reports, "The makers of antacids such as Prilosec® want them to believe that they are too acidic, when in reality it is not that they are too acidic but HCl deficient. If they have been deficient for a long time, they probably have an ulcer. Once they address the ulcer, they can fix the problem, which was too little acid, by adding Zypan®."

What Else Causes Stomach Ulcers?

In addition to lack of HCl, the long-term overuse of antacids is one of the reasons why many people suffer from ulcers.

Other common causes of stomach ulcers include the use of tobacco, coffee, alcohol, nutrient deficiencies and stress.

Author Earl Mindell writes that it is now estimated that up to one-third of all bleeding ulcers are caused by taking nonsteroidal anti-inflammatory drugs (NSAIDs) such as Aspirin® and Ibuprofen®. These drugs relieve pain, but at a cost. NSAIDs cause gastrointestinal discomfort which indicates that damage is occurring. However, by the time the stomach is in pain, massive damage has occurred. In many cases, the antacids and H2 blockers given to alleviate the symptoms of stomach pain mask the symptoms until the problem is life threatening.[19]

All of these medications simply deal with symptoms, not the cause. A better approach is to identify the causes of ulcers.

Dr. Murray writes that a possible cause of ulcers could be food allergies. A diet eliminating food allergies may help to treat and prevent ulcers. He recommends avoiding milk products which, while they may seem soothing, may aggravate the ulcer. He also recommends avoiding wheat and soy, which are common allergens.[20]

An extremely popular natural alternative for treating an ulcer is drinking cabbage juice. It appears to increase the amount of protective substances that line the intestinal wall. I highly recommend that you work with your health professional for help with stomach ulcers.

What About Gas?

We are taught two things about gas. Everyone has it, and there's nothing we can do about it! Both are wrong.

Most of my clients know that the first cause of gas is the lack of HCl, so I commonly suggest they take Zypan®, or another enzyme containing HCl with meals.

Anything that hinders your body's ability to digest food causes excess gas; especially foods that are more difficult to digest, or more processed, such as junk foods, fried foods and foods containing white sugar and white flour.

Candida yeast creates a waste product that creates gas symptoms. Common symptoms of overgrowth of this yeast are: Vaginal discharge, fungus, itching under the skin, and brain fog. (See your health professional for help with this.)

Combining the wrong types of foods at one meal can also cause gas. If you have ever eaten at a buffet and ended up with incredible gas or bloating, then this is what has happened. For example, eating fruit after a protein/starch meal can cause gas.

Anxiety, stress, emotional upsets and simply eating too fast can also cause gas. Overeating, some drugs and antibiotics are also possible culprits.

And finally, I recommend checking for parasites. I think everyone should do a parasite cleanse at least once a year whether you travel overseas or not. Your health care professional can order a stool test for parasites. (Wormwood Complex by MediHerb® is a natural herbal formula which is great for eliminating parasites. MediHerb® is distributed in the United States by Standard Process® and is only sold through health professionals.)

Excessive gas may, however, be a symptom of more serious problems with the colon, such as diverticulitis. If these solutions don't help, see your doctor.

How Did These Problems Begin?

Improper digestion is linked to every disease, from acne to arthritis. These problems may even begin as early as infancy. If your mother ate a good diet and nursed you with mother's milk, you were given an excellent opportunity for great digestion. If she wasn't so careful, then you might have had stomach problems as a baby, such as colic or throwing up what you were fed, which many parents and pediatricians consider normal.

You probably know by now that it's not normal, but it is common! I've had frantic moms call me for help with their newborn babies. I recommended a digestive enzyme be put in their milk and the colic left. Even babies need enzymes sometimes!

Many children acquire stomach problems before their first birthday! Our stomachs weren't created to digest ice cream, soda and candy as kids are eating them today. Mom's regularly give their children foods that we shouldn't even eat!

The other day I heard of a woman who was putting soda in her baby's bottle! It may be a few years, but in time this child will have serious digestive problems due to the maldigestion of protein, fats or carbohydrates. It's just a matter of time.

If You Can't Breast Feed

According to nutritionist Dr. Donna Smith, infants need only mother's milk for their first 12 months to develop strong digestive systems from a mother who is eating 90% or more of only natural food as outlined in this book. If the mother is unable to breast feed, she should feed her infant only goat's milk (which is the closest to mother's milk).

Digestion Tips

For more help with digestion, you'll want to read Part 5 about designing your life for health where I review a clinical program for improving your digestion and health.

Let's move on to the next part of your check-up, and see how remarkable your liver is for great health.

Chapter Four

Your Liver Is Your Major Fat-Burning Organ

Feeling lousy? Did you know that a great part of your health depends on your liver—especially weight loss and fatigue!

Your liver is the largest gland in your body, and to many nutritionists, it's one of the most important glands. I remember reading that in China, when they greet you, they are actually asking how your health is regarding the state of your liver and digestion! It's the only organ that will regenerate itself if part of it becomes damaged, and your body can't function without it.

In the front of this book, I gave a few testimonies from my clients who have helped themselves by cleansing their livers. They slept better, lost weight, lowered their cholesterol and eliminated headaches.

The functions of the liver are involved in the majority of health problems that I see daily. The more I study the liver, the more I am amazed at what it does. Research shows that the liver performs more than 500 different functions. A clean liver will produce natural antihistimines for high immunity, cleanse the blood, help the body to burn fat, and help maintain hormone balance.

The liver helps to regulate thyroid function by converting T4, thyroxine to T3, triodothyronine. So a dysfunctional liver can be involved in hypothyroidism, and later, weight gain that is difficult to lose until you cleanse your liver.

The liver breaks down or metabolizes hormones such as estrogen, testosterone, cortisol, adrenaline, and insulin. For example, some symptoms of PMS and menopause may occur because the liver is congested.

Sugars not needed for immediate energy are stored in the liver. Excess food is converted to fat in the liver and then moved to the fatty tissues of the body for storage. That's why most diets for weight loss and lowering cholesterol are doomed to fail if cleansing the liver isn't involved.

So to summarize, your liver helps your thyroid, hormone balance, blood-sugar levels, and fat-burning or cholesterol-lowering efforts! Let's give the liver some respect!

In this chapter, we'll focus on the liver's role as a fat-burner and toxin filter.

The Liver As a Fat Burner

Most people are unaware about how their liver works, so they don't see any connection between the earlier listed toxins, liver health and weight loss.

In an ideal situation, your liver would pump excess fat out of the body through bile into the small intestines. However, as I've said throughout this book, few Americans have an ideal situation!

Anyone with problems such as weight gain, a pot belly, cellulite, high cholesterol and high triglycerides, to name a few, has a problem with how fats are metabolized and eliminated. As I learned from Dr. Michael Dobbins, a chiropractor who practices in Alameda, California and who teaches seminars about nutrition to doctors around the country, weight issues are all "liver" issues.

If the liver is sluggish or toxic, due to a high toxic load, it's harder to remove the fat that circulates in the bloodstream, allowing fat to build up in the blood vessels, liver, and eventually other tissues. It also gets deposited in such areas as your hips, thighs and bottom!

Uh-Oh, My Liver Is Too Fat!

After years and years of eating the typical American diet, most Americans begin to gain weight, without even trying! What's been happening is that year after year, the liver is getting more toxic and fatter, which is referred to as a "fatty" liver. However, you probably don't even know this is happening as this condition is quite common and most doctors don't consider it very serious.

How would you know if your liver is sluggish, toxic or even fatty? Here are some health symptoms that can result from a sluggish, toxic or fatty liver:

Symptoms of a Sluggish, Fatty Liver

- Depression
- Great fatigue
- Reflux
- PMS
- Constipation
- Diarrhea
- Dry skin
- Itchy skin
- Gallstones
- Bloating
- Sugar cravings
- Hypoglycemia
- Irritability/anger
- Hot flashes
- Candida
- Cellulite
- Allergies
- Body odor
- Acne
- Bad breath
- Edema
- Unexplained weight gain
- Poor digestion and heartburn
- Food and chemical sensitivities
- Menopausal symptoms
- Nausea
- Dry mouth
- Liver spots
- Hemorrhoids
- Gallbladder disease
- Hormone imbalance
- Diabetes
- Brain fog
- Headaches
- High cholesterol
- High-blood pressure
- Cirrhosis
- Skin rashes
- Fibromyalgia
- Chronic Fatigue Snydrome
- Joint pain
- Autoimmune diseases

Producing Bile is Vital

The liver secretes bile, a fluid stored in the gallbladder for release when needed in digestion. Bile is necessary for the digestion of fats and also assists in the absorption of fat-soluble vitamins A, D, E, F, and K, and helps assimilate calcium. Bile helps promote peristalsis, the wavelike movement of the colon, to prevent constipation. Problems with this function can include a toxic gallbladder, gallstones, or clogged bile ducts.

Common Symptoms of Bile Problems

- Light colored stools
- Belching
- Constipation
- Problems digesting fats
- Hormone imbalance
- Gas and bloating
- Pain over the gallbladder
- Dry skin
- Weight gain

We need some good fats and even cholesterol so our body can produce hormones, nourish our skin, and for normal metabolism for weight and fat loss.

A deficiency of bile can hinder fat digestion and weight loss. According to nutritionist and author of *The Fat Flush Plan,* Ann Louise Gittleman, bile is the key to the liver's ability to digest and assimilate fats. The lack of proper nutrients, congestion, or even clogged bile ducts can hamper bile flow and result in less bile production. If there is not enough bile produced, fat cannot be emulsified or broken down.[21]

What About Gallbladder Flushes

A common "fix" is an olive oil flush. Here's what nutritionist Dr. Dobbins says about liver/gallbladder flushes:

"I don't recommend that people do olive oil purges. I suggest that they take more time and cleanse the liver/gallbladder more gradually. If there is a stone, it may be crystalline in composition and have sharp edges. Aggressively moving such a stone through the bile duct may cause bleeding. It doesn't necessarily have to be removed since not all stones cause problems. You can achieve the same results with the cleanses in this book. So don't force it; your body is smarter than you. Sometimes we just need to trust the body's healing and wisdom. Restore balance to the endocrine system and get the liver and thyroid working properly."

I used to have my clients do a purge until I started using the cleanse in this book. I've even had people call me from the phone book, who are are in severe pain because they didn't even know how to do it properly. My assistant, Anne, went to a doctor once who encouraged her to do a gallbladder cleanse, and then told her not to call him if she ended up in the Emergency Room at the hospital! So she didn't do it.

If you feel you may have gallbladder problems, see your health care professional. If you've had your gallbladder removed, it's vital that you don't "eat everything you want." Your ability to metabolize fat, and produce hormones is compromised. **Realize it could take 6 months and even a year for you to help your liver burn fat and lose weight.** Your health care professional can determine what type of ongoing supplementation you will need.

How Fiber Lowers Cholesterol Levels

Fiber is vital for liver health because the bile that the liver makes is recycled, except when you eat fiber. Fiber produces a gel-like coating inside the intestines that prevents the bile from being absorbed and reused. So the bile is flushed out of the body, along with toxins and fat. Now the liver makes bile again, but the liver needs cholesterol for this process. So it takes cholesterol from the blood stream and blood cholesterol levels drop. This is why fiber lowers cholesterol levels and is so vital in preventing heart disease and circulatory disorders.

Dr. Jonathan Wright, in his book, *Dr. Wright's Guide to Healing With Nutrition,* states that gallbladder attacks could be completely avoided by eliminating allergenic foods from the diet. Dr. Wright reports that he hasn't had to refer anyone for gallbladder surgery since 1979. He must be on to something![22]

The Liver As a Blood Filter of Toxins

The liver is a major filter for impurities in the blood. Here is a list of things it has to break down and eliminate.

Common Toxins

• Chemicals	• Drugs	• Alcohol
• Hormones	• Allergens	• Bacteria
• Pesticides	• Herbicides	• Medications
• Food additives	• Metals	

The healthier the liver, the quicker these toxins will be eliminated from the body.

I first learned about liver detoxification from Dr. Michael Dobbins. He explained that our livers are always cleansing or detoxifying our blood, all day, every day of our lives. (What hard workers!) Most of the liver's "detoxification" or cleansing process involves two different phases, called Phase 1 and Phase 2 detoxification pathways. (Phase 1 is called the Cytochrome P450 system and Phase 2 is called conjugation, but all you really need to know is that these pathways are vital for good health and fat loss!)

Here's what this means in simple terms: During these phases, the liver changes harmful toxins into unharmful, water-soluble substances so the kidneys and intestines can eliminate them. When these organs are inefficient, internal cleansing is impaired, and so is fat-burning and many other important functions of the liver.

Enzymes in the first phase of cleansing begin the process of detoxifying substances such as medications and chemicals. Unfortunately, during this process, free radicals are generated. That's where the second phase comes in. The second phase helps eliminate toxins through the urine or bile.

While these processes sound complex, they depend on simple nutrition. For example, according to Dr. Michael Dobbins, foods such as broccoli, brussels sprouts, cabbage, garlic, and red pepper help the liver to do its thing!

I've written an extensive list of foods that will keep your liver healthy in chapter 6 and we'll get to the liver cleanse in chapter 7.

What Liver Tests Reveal

Many of my overweight clients who have come to see me have blood test results from their doctors. According to the medical interpretation of their liver tests (SGOT, SGPT, alkaline phosphatase or bilirubin tests), there was absolutely no liver dysfunction. The purpose for these tests is to check liver enzymes so they can spot elevations that can occur when the liver cells rupture. However, according to author of *The Mysterious Cause of All Illness,* Dr. Jon Matsen, these tests don't pick up early-stage liver overload.[23]

These tests are checking late-stage liver disease; they don't determine liver function or overload. At this point, though, it's a bit late!

A routine symptom survey that I run in my office shows that many people have an overloaded, sluggish liver. In fact Dr. Matsen believes that even people without the obvious symptoms may have an overloaded liver (fatigue, mood swings, PMS, irritability, and water retention).[24]

I've heard Dr. Bond say, "If you've lived in America for more than 10 years, you need to cleanse your liver!"

I would add to that, if you are having trouble lowering your cholesterol or triglycerides, losing weight, or have excess sweating or hot flashes, then you need to cleanse your liver! There is probably a lot of fat that has infiltrated into your liver that can be gradually removed through a liver cleanse. Only when this is achieved, will you achieve your goal! The program outlined in chapter 7 will show you exactly how to improve your liver function.

The liver is so amazing! Here's another testimony from a client named Sue who struggled for years with feeling extremely hot with excessive sweating and was helped with a liver product:

"I can't believe after 5 years of misery, that it's this simple! With a history of drugs and shots, I have been miserable. After two days, I began to feel normal again! And now I actually even experience being cool!"

What Else Hurts the Liver?

Besides the toxic load, what else can cause a sluggish or toxic liver?

In addition to toxins and medications, many of the foods that we grew up eating hinder the liver's function. So when you get to chapter 7, don't think of it as foods that are being taken away from you. Think of it as eliminating foods that are hindering your liver!

Foods and Factors That Hurt Your Liver

- Fried foods and saturated fats
- Foods made from white flour
- Foods which contain white sugar
- A diet high in red meat
- Hydrogenated oils and trans fats
- Alcohol
- Bowel toxicity or leaky gut
- Pharmaceutical medications
- Anabolic steroids
- Excessive refined carbohydrates
- Overeating
- Eating large meals at night
- Pork and shellfish
- High-fat dairy products
- Hair colors and dyes
- Excess sun
- Candida overgrowth
- Oral contraceptives
- Caffeine

Do You Have Syndrome X?

Recently, you might have heard about Syndrome X, which refers to high levels of circulating insulin. People with Syndrome X usually have high levels of blood fats, such as triglycerides and LDL. Writers, such as the authors of the book *Sugar Busters,* believe that high levels of insulin are an even more important indicator of heart disease than high levels of cholesterol.[25]

The problem with high levels of insulin is that insulin is a fat-storing hormone. So people with Syndrome X usually have more of a chance of having high blood fats, a fatty liver and weight gain.

What causes Syndrome X? Eating processed foods for many years, such as refined carbohydrates, sugars and the wrong fats. In order to help your liver, then, you will want to follow the dietary guidelines in this book to help you lower insulin levels and thus support your liver as a fat-burning organ. A client named Mary couldn't follow my cleanse because of her high insulin levels. So she ate protein and vegetables for a week, to lower her insulin levels which cut sugar cravings. Then I suggested she follow the cleanse in chapter 7. (Ask your doctor for a check of your insulin level.)

What About High-Protein Diets and the Liver?

You and I have met people who have lost weight and fat following a high-protein diet. Yet many people get even fatter, or nothing happened! Why?

These diets help with weight loss because they reduce insulin levels. So a person with a fairly healthy liver usually burns fat. But a person who follows a high-protein diet and has a compromised or fatty liver, will just gain fat!

Even people who do lose weight can gain it all back again if the liver is never addressed. I've found that unless you improve liver function, these diets can increase the workload of the liver, causing you to store more fat.

What About Drugs and Your Liver?

My clients are usually unaware of the damaging effect of many medications on their liver.

So often clients tell me that they are taking some type of drug for their symptoms when the reason they need the drug is really a nutritional one. A common example is taking a drug for leg cramps which is often a deficiency in either calcium, magnesium, Vitamin B complex or Vitamin E complex.

Are You Deficient in Aspirin®?

If you have a headache, your doctor will prescribe Aspirin®. Your headache will usually disappear. But no one asks about what might have caused the headache. Looking at the treatment, you could conclude the headache was caused by an Aspirin deficiency!

Dr. Joel Robbins, a friend and practicing chiropractor in Tulsa, shares an interesting perspective on how drugs work in his book, *Health Through Nutrition*.[26] He explains,

> Aspirin will relieve any pain in the body, from a headache to a toe ache—except for a stomachache. Why? Every Aspirin (buffered or not) causes a teaspoon worth of bleeding in the digestive tract. If you have a headache, and you take an Aspirin causing internal bleeding, which do you think would be more life threatening? In most cases the internal bleeding. The body must now shift its attention to the higher priority problem (the stomach), giving the appearance that the headache disappeared. Did the Aspirin remove the cause of the headache? Not at all, it just created a more life-threatening situation.

Dr. Donna Smith gives a practical example of this: "You've heard the joke about the man who is complaining non-stop about the pain in his thumb when all of a sudden a heavy object falls on his big toe, and now he no longer feels any pain in his thumb. The body turned off the thumb pain signal to communicate to you the new toe pain."

If the Aspirin doesn't take away the headache, it just means that the internal bleeding in your stomach is not more life threatening than what is causing your headache.

(By the way, there are many causes for headaches. Chronic headaches may be due to allergies, a sluggish liver, a toxic bloodstream, or the previous use of caffeine, soda or sugar. As I've seen in my practice, headaches are often easily eliminated with a change in diet. It's better to find and correct the cause once and for all instead of continually using pain killers such as Aspirin. Your natural health professional can help you.)

Why doesn't Aspirin take care of stomach pain? The stomach pain means your body's attention is already focused on the stomach. Additional stress to the stomach such as internal bleeding caused by taking an Aspirin will not force the body to shift its attention elsewhere in the body; thus the pain remains in the stomach.

You might wonder about Tylenol®. Does Tylenol really eliminate stomach pain? No, what it does is it **alleviates stomach pain by harming the liver,** causing the body to move its attention from the stomach to the liver, thus giving the false impression that it cured the stomach pain.

According to nutritionist Dr. Linda Rector Page, Americans take over 85 million Aspirins every day! It's become part of our lives, so much so that we don't even think of it as a drug. But even Aspirin can hurt you. She links ringing in the ears and gastrointestinal problems as early signs of Aspirin overdose. Long-term Aspirin users are at higher risk for gastric bleeding. Buffered or enteric coated Aspirin is just as likely as regular Aspirin to cause gastric bleeding.[27]

Dr. Joel Robbins explains that with few exceptions, all drugs work in a similar fashion as the Aspirin. On the other hand, if the drug is not more life threatening than the symptom for which it is taken, the drug will not produce symptomatic relief; thus a more life-threatening drug will have to be taken to get relief. When the body focuses on the drug you become symptom free; yet in most cases the cause isn't eliminated. No healing took place.

Taking drugs costs in other ways, too. One client brought in a drug which had the following label: "These pills are expensive. Take them only as often as you can afford to!"

How Do Drugs Hurt the Liver?

It's well known that Acetaminophen (Tylenol®) can cause liver damage. But according to health writer and researcher Dr. Bruce West, it seems as though pain killers do more than kill pain.

In his *Health Alert,* he reports that Tylenol® taken with just three alcoholic drinks can poison your liver. So can overdosing with Tylenol® or using it in conjunction with other cold and flu remedies. Acetaminophen is the active ingredient in many drugs. In this article, Dr. West recommends that if you frequently use any of the following drugs, have your doctor test your liver: Tylenol®, Excedrin®, Percocet®, Vicodin®, Sinutab®, Sudafed®, 4-Way Cold®, Bayer Select Flu Relief®, Benedryl

Cold®, Comtrex Hot Flu Relief®, Dristan Cold and Flu®, Nyquil Liquicaps®, Robitussin Honey Flu®, Tylenol Cold and Flu®, Vicks Dayquil Liquicaps®, Aspirin-Free Excedrin Caplets®, Anacin-3®, Children's Tylenol Cold®, Dorcol Children's Fever and Pain Reducer®, Feverall Children's®, Infants' Anacin-3®, Tylenol Children's Elixir®, St. Joseph's Aspirin-Free Fever Reducer for Children®.[28]

He also says that Acetaminophen overdoses are a bigger cause of liver failure than prescription drugs recently banned for liver poisoning—like the diabetes drug, Rezulin®. Dr. West says that if you have any kind of liver problem, stay away from these pain killers. If you choose to use any drug with Acetaminophen, experts suggest you limit your daily Acetaminophen intake to the amount in four extra-strength pills or two grams total from all medicines.[29]

I highly recommend that you read about the side effects of any drugs you are currently taking in a PDR (Physician Desk Reference), and see what it is costing you in other areas of your body. Look up every drug that you take—even, "safe, over-the-counter" drugs. (After reading this chapter, you might wonder if there is such a thing!)

In chapter 7, you'll see that even arthritis and osteoporosis pain can be treated naturally.

What Can I Do?

One of the best things you can do to support your liver is to get plenty of exercise and eat a clean, healthy diet high in organic vegetables, fruit and protein and low in refined, processed foods and saturated fats.

Additionally, I highly recommend the cleanse program listed in chapter 7 in this book. I would recommend that you work with a natural health care professional while you follow this program.

After the liver breaks down toxins, they must be eliminated through your urine and bowel movements. So healthy colon function is the next part of your tune-up.

Chapter Five

Are You Sure You're Not Constipated?

Have you ever noticed that when we're young, we look for cereals that are fun and tasty, but after we hit 40 or 50, we are happy to trade in the plastic toys for a cereal that contains lots of fiber!

A client named Wendy said, "I used to feel like my abdomen was a rock; after following the cleanse that Lorrie recommended, it's back to normal. I'm so excited! I can't believe that no one tells us how to cleanse our colon, or what to use."

More than 45 million Americans use laxatives, and at least a fifth of these people use them weekly. Laxatives, which contain stimulants, irritate the intestinal tract. Long term, this causes poor muscle tone and dependence on laxatives.

In the previous chapters, we've seen the importance of a healthy stomach and liver for proper digestion, health and weight loss. Additionally, a deficiency of three major factors can contribute to bowel problems and poor health:

1. **Fiber**
2. **Friendly bacteria**
3. **Essential fats**

In this chapter, we'll look at how all three of these nutrients contribute to good health, starting with fiber.

Processed, fiberless foods are like paste on your intestinal wall. Without fiber, this "paste" has nothing to move it out. I remember as a young girl, stirring up a mixture of flour and water to make a paste for a school project. Every time I think of white flour products, I remember the consistency of this paste. It's similar to the stuff that clings to the walls of the intestines when we don't have enough fiber to keep things moving.

More About Fiber

Fiber is the indigestible remnant in fruits, vegetables, nuts, seeds, beans, peas and whole grains that is not broken down. Fiber is found mainly in plant-based foods; animal foods like meat, fish, poultry and dairy do not have fiber.

Fiber acts like a broom sweeping through the digestive system, gently absorbing water and other materials while sweeping toxins, fats and waste material through the colon. This is how you lose weight!

The average American consumes only 7 to 10 grams of dietary fiber, and that's on a good day! The National Cancer Institute, American Cancer Society and American Heart Association recommend that we increase our fiber intake from 10 grams to 35-40. People in some third-world countries who experience much lower rates of disease ingest almost four times more fiber than we do—getting 60 to even 100 grams per day. That's a lot of time in the bathroom!

A typical American diet is a low-fiber diet that consists of meat, white bread, pancakes made with white flour, peanut butter and jelly on white bread, French fries, and few, if any, vegetables. You've probably heard the government statistic that less than 5% of Americans get their recommended servings of fruits and vegetables, all good sources of natural fiber.

We need both soluble and insoluble fibers. Without enough fiber, the walls of the colon can accumulate toxins. In fact many people have as much as 10 pounds of old waste in their bowels, according to Dr. Bernard Jensen in his book, *Tissue Cleansing Through Bowel Management.* Dr. Jensen also says:

In the 50 years I've spent helping people to overcome illness, disability, and disease, it has become crystal clear that poor bowel management lies at the root of most people's health problems.[30]

You'll learn more about the benefits of fiber and how to get it in the next two chapters of this book. Let's now look at toxins and how they affect the colon.

Toxins Linked to Disease

Dr. Jensen taught that disease starts in the colon. When the eliminative channels are underactive, toxins accumulate in the colon and later back up into the liver and kidneys.

You might understand how accumulated toxins in the body can cause such problems as headaches, constipation, skin problems and weight gain, but according to Dr. Jensen, it's also linked to serious problems such as arthritis, cancer and degenerative autoimmune conditions.

Both British and South African medical scientists strongly insist that what is usually referred to as "regularity" may be a matter of life and death. Insufficient numbers of bowel movements and too little fiber and bulk in the feces may often explain the existence of gall bladder disorders, heart problems, varicose veins, appendicitis, clotting in deep veins, hiatal hernia, diverticulosis, arthritis and cancer of the colon. This complete turn-around in medical orientation comes from top-notch surgeons and biochemists.[31]

Dr. Jensen further explained the link of colon health to heart problems. He reported that retaining feces is linked to heart disorders, as the removal of fiber from the diet raises serum cholesterol levels and predisposes the body to coronary disease. He believed that the removal of fiber from the diet is also responsible for tumors and cancer due to biochemical changes associated with poor bowel elimination.[32]

Where Does It Go?

Where does waste that cannot be eliminated go? It's estimated that between 4-25 pounds of waste can accumulate on the colon wall! Some of it builds up on the colon walls (impacted feces, dead tissue, mucus, and parasites) and the rest may even block the digestive tract. When the eliminative channels are sluggish, waste is forced to come out through the skin which explains how a sluggish liver/colon can cause skin problems. Uh-oh!

Imagine what your kitchen would be like if you just kept dumping garbage into sacks, but you never took out the garbage! Well, imagine what your colon is like when toxins are not eliminated.

I like how Dr. Lindsey Duncan, a practicing Certified Nutritionist in California puts it: "If you are eating three meals a day, and eliminating once, where are the other two meals?"[33]

The two meals are still in your colon, waiting for some enzymes, fiber and water to push them along! Most people think that "being regular" is having one bowel movement a day. But less than 2-3 bowel movements a day is a sign of constipation. And constipation may be a warning sign of other more serious problems in the stomach, liver, or thyroid. If you've only had a few bowel movements a week, dozens of meals are still in your colon, unless you've done something to eliminate them.

Breast-fed babies are good examples of good digestion; after they eat, they immediately eliminate. We should, too.

Recently a female client named Sharon used some of my products to cleanse her colon. Sharon reported, "After a few days, I saw kernels of corn being eliminated in my stools. The surprising thing was that I realized it had been nearly a month since I had eaten any corn!"

In addition to being toxic, impacted waste hinders absorption of nutrients through the intestinal wall. You may be taking supplements, and even eating healthy foods with good nutrition in them, but if your intestinal wall is hindered from absorption because of damage from toxins, (or fecal impactions along the intestinal wall), you may not be absorbing what you eat! Accumulation of toxins in the colon is also a breeding ground for parasites, viruses, yeast and types of bacteria that are considered unfriendly.

Let's look at the second factor important for good bowel health.

Howdy!

There are two types of bacteria living in your colon: Friendly and unfriendly. Friendly bacteria help break up food so the small villi which line the intestines can absorb it. The average intestine contains more than 500 species of beneficial, friendly bacteria. The most common are lactobacillus acidophilus and bifidobacterium bifidus. These friendly bacteria also act as a natural antibiotic.

Because both types of bacteria have their functions, the balance of these bacteria is vital. Your colon should have at least 85% healthy, friendly (lactobacillus) and 15% unfriendly (coliform) bacteria. Unfortunately, the average colon contains the opposite! When the balance of friendly to unfriendly bacteria is compromised, health problems begin. What hurts the good bacteria: Sugar, stress, chlorinated water, processed foods and the use of antibiotics, to name a few.

According to cancer expert Dr. Patrick Quillin, author of *Beating Cancer With Nutrition*, friendly bacteria are vital. Here is a list of what these good guys do:[34]

Benefits of Friendly Bacteria

- They help your body fight against harmful bacteria, viruses and yeast.
- They stimulate the function of your immune system.
- They help your body produce essential vitamins.
- They protect the gut mucosa.
- They improve the pH of the colon.
- They aid in the digestion and absorption of nutrients.
- They reduce the carcinogenic by-products.

People who have taken many antibiotics often lose the balance of friendly bacteria because the antibiotics kill both the friendly (good) and unfriendly (bad) bacteria. If you have taken antibiotics, you may have compromised your intestinal bacteria balance, and you will need to replace this bacteria by taking an acidophilus supplement. I recommend Lact-Enz® and/or Zymex® by Standard Process®. These products are great support for people with irritable bowel syndrome (IBS). Additionally, your health professional can recommend herbs to help your intestines re-establish friendly bacteria.

Now we'll look at the third vital factor for colon health.

Essential Fats

Essential fatty acids are vital for healthy cell membranes and healthy liver and colon function. Additionally, they help improve the functioning of the entire digestive tract, helping to avoid gas and constipation.

Sources of these "good" essential fats include cold-water fish, such as mackerel, salmon, tuna and trout. Flaxseed oil is a great plant source of essential fat, either taken by the teaspoon or in capsules.

Since these oils can become rancid quickly, know your source. I learned from Dr. Janet Lang, (See pages 40-41.) that not all flax supplements are alike. Some companies try to hide the rancid taste by "deodorizing" the oils. That's why they should be cold-pressed, come in a dark bottle, be kept refrigerated, and have an expiration date. She recommends that you taste the oil or bite one of the capsules open with your teeth. If it tastes very bitter, it's rancid.

Fresh flax oil should have a pleasant nutty flavor. You can purchase fresh flaxseeds and grind them up in a coffee grinder to use as a great source of fiber. (I use Standard Process Linum B6 flaxseed oil which you can order from your natural healthcare professional.)

Answer on the First Ring!

A client named Joan didn't like to use public restrooms. She told me, "It was common for me to hold it until I got home, repeatedly ignoring the urge to eliminate." I told her that when Nature calls, you must answer on the first ring! Otherwise, sooner or later, your body won't be able to respond appropriately. Eventually symptoms occur such as the ones on the list below:

Constipation or diarrhea, poor digestion, chronic yeast infections, depressed immune system, weight problems, acne, arthritis, asthma, allergies, cold sores, insomnia, irritability, poor circulation, skin disorders, mood swings, low sex drive, short term memory problems, sleeping problems, urinary tract infections, apathy, fatigue, gas, bloating, confusion, lower backache, body odor, bad breath, and depression.

Following the suggestions in this chapter and book will help you improve liver, digestive and colon function, thus improving all of these symptoms without the use of drugs.

What Else Hurts the Colon?

* White bread and refined foods
* Milk and milk products
* Regular use of antibiotics
* Consistent overeating
* Prescription drugs
* Over-cooked food
* B complex deficiency
* Stress
* Lack of sufficient water
* Lack of exercise

Diseases of the Colon

It's surprising what can happen to the colon without fiber, essential fat, and friendly bacteria. While the cleanse described in this book will help you somewhat, you'll want to work with your natural health care professional if you have any of the following problems.

* Ulcers of the bowel can occur due to infections or irritations in the muscle tissue. It can result in open sores, bleeding and pain.

* Spastic or irritable bowel can have symptoms of constipation and diarrhea and aching or sharp pains.

* Crohn's Disease is a severe inflammatory reaction that can affect any portion of the GI tract.

• Colitis is an irritable bowel condition that is related to emotional stress. Fear, stress and worry can upset the delicate tissues of the body.

• Diverticular diseases happen when the diet lacks fiber and the colonic muscle forces feces through the colon. The weak muscle tissue forms a small pouch or hernia. Feces can accumulate within these sacs or pouches which can become infected and inflamed.

What Is a Leaky Gut?

The intestinal wall is coated with hundreds of different types of microorganisms, both friendly and unfriendly bacteria. This coating works with the physical lining of the intestinal tract to provide a protective filter. It filters out damaging substances, such as toxins, undigested food, and unfriendly bacteria. It also allows nutrients, digested food, and water to go into circulation. This is good.

However, bad dietary and bowel habits can cause a breakdown of this protective lining, creating openings where substances (toxins, undigested foods, drugs) that were not supposed to pass through the lining do so and then get into the bloodstream. (How would you ever know?) This isn't good!

As the lining becomes damaged, it allows passage of more toxins into circulation. This is called "leaky gut," and it has been clinically linked to inflammatory joint disease, food allergies and intolerances.

According to authors DeAnn Liska and Dan Lukaczer, in a review article of the *Journal of the American Nutraceutical Association,* the factors that cause leaky gut include:[35]

What Causes a Leaky Gut?

• Premature birth	• Corticosteroids
• Gastrointestinal infections	• Excessive stress
• Cancer radiation therapy	• NSAIDs
• Nutrient deficiencies	• Fasting
• Alcohol	• Food allergies

• Excessive simple sugar consumption

• Whole food exposure prior to 4-6 months of age

The overuse of antibiotics, the growth of unfriendly bacteria and nonsteroidal, anti-inflammatory drugs (NSAIDS) such as Ibuprofen® and Aspirin® damage the gut lining.[36] Surprisingly, people with an inflammatory joint disease are often prescribed NSAIDs for pain relief which further causes more problems!

It's possible to heal a leaky gut. You'll want to work with your natural health care professional for special dietary suggestions and nutritional supplements.

Having a healthy colon is vital! Below are diseases associated with food allergies and intolerances.[37]

System	Symptoms/Disease
Gastrointestinal	Canker sores, celiac disease, chronic diarrhea, stomach ulcers, duodenal ulcers, recurrent mouth ulcers, indigestion, nausea, vomiting, constipation, gas, gastritis, irritable bowel syndrome, malabsorption, ulcerative colitis Crohn's disease, colic (babies)
Genitourinary	Bed wetting, chronic bladder infections, nephrotic syndrome, frequent urination
Immune	Serious otitis media
Mental/Emotional	Attention deficit disorder, depression, anxiety, memory loss, epileptic seizures, schizophrenia
Musculoskeletal	Joint pain, myalgias, rheumatoid arthritis
Respiratory	Asthma, chronic or allergic sinusitis, constant runny nose or congested nose, nasal polyps
Cardiovascular	Irregular heart rhythm, vasculitis, inflammation of the veins producing purpura, spontaneous bruising, urticaria, edema
Skin	Eczema, psoriasis, urticaria, red itchy eyes, itchy skin
Miscellaneous	Migraine headaches

So good health is connected to the stomach, liver, and colon! My, where do I begin!

Follow an "internal" cleanse which will deal with every part of your digestion and assist the process of healing throughout your body.

Let's now look at the many, many benefits of cleansing.

PART FOUR

Why Should I Cleanse?

Chapter Six

What Are the Benefits of Cleansing?

It's amazing to me how Americans spend hours cleaning their cars, homes, and other belongings. They routinely take out the garbage, wash the car and do laundry. But when was the last time they cleaned their colon, liver or bloodstream? Most people say, "Never!" No wonder they feel lousy!

We routinely take care of our hair, skin, and teeth, but we rarely pay attention to the most important parts of the human body: The stomach, liver, colon, kidney, lymphatic system and bloodstream. These parts are irreplaceable. Imagine though, if we could take them in for cleansing after every 1,000 miles or so—drop them off on Friday and pick them up on Tuesday!

No, so far there aren't any "liver washaterias," or "colon laundromatics." But we can just do it ourselves, in the privacy of our own homes! Again, think of it as taking a shower on the inside!

I encourage every client to do an "internal" cleanse and often tell them the benefits at their first appointment. However, when I talk to my clients about internal body cleansing, it seems like the same couple of questions come up. People will ask me if they can grow back a head of hair (usually not!) or change their hair color from gray to their natural color (rarely!) However, it's still worth the effort and time to cleanse!

So what will cleansing do for you? **Weight loss, lower cholesterol, more energy!** If you've been trying to lose weight and keep gaining and regaining the same pounds, you need to cleanse. Cleansing will help your liver burn fat instead of store fat. Cleansing helps the liver become a fat-burning organ. But it also helps with any other condition of excess fat, as in high triglycerides or high cholesterol.

Because toxins can be stored in any organ or tissue of your body, cleansing and eliminating toxins can affect you mentally, emotionally and physically. For example, eliminating toxins in the brain can help you think more clearly. Eliminating toxins in the liver can improve any hormone imbalance, male or female. Cleansing will help eliminate body odor and bad breath as well. The benefits are often terrific.

Let's look at a general list of the many benefits of cleansing I've compiled from Dr. Bruce Bond and observed in my professional nutritional practice.

Benefits of Cleansing

- Improved digestion and elimination
- Improved and easier weight loss
- Improved physical appearance
- Decreased cravings and addictions
- Cleanse and purify bloodstream
- Improved sleep
- Increased muscle tone
- Increased stamina
- Eliminate body odor
- Eliminate headaches
- Reduction in risk of many diseases
- More positive outlook on life
- Feel happier and healthier
- Break the cycle of overeating
- Break desire for artificial sweets
- Help normalize your metabolism
- Deal with stress more effectively
- Lower your blood pressure
- Increased energy
- Stronger immune system
- Normal appetite
- Improved circulation
- Better concentration/focus
- Clearer skin
- Greater health
- Eliminate bad breath
- Eliminate mouth sores
- Clearer eyes
- Eliminate allergies
- Look better in your clothes
- Retrain your taste buds
- Feel more motivated
- Improve your skin
- Help slow down aging
- Lower your cholesterol
- Be more productive

What Happens When You Cleanse?

Internal cleansing is one of the most powerful natural healing therapies there is. Cleansing helps us correct damage done to us by our diet and lifestyle. It's an ancient remedy that can correct literally hundreds of health concerns.

I began cleansing more than 30 years ago, and I feel it's one of the most important parts of my health routine and the reason I've been successful in keeping off the weight that I lost twenty years ago. I always cleanse a minimum of twice a year.

I'm always surprised at what happens to me personally when I cleanse. Old habits quickly fall away. For example, I do, on occasion, enjoy a "good" cup of coffee. Yet it's surprising to me how coffee doesn't even taste good when I finish my cleanse. My energy always increases, any fatigue or aches completely disappear, and I feel more creative! My sleep is sounder and I notice no symptoms of hormone imbalance.

During the process of cleansing, your body breaks down stored chemicals in the blood and throughout the body. Every cell can more easily repair itself and eliminate its waste. Cleansing always improves the process of elimination and assists the release of toxins from the colon, kidney, liver, lungs, spleen, bladder, skin and lymphatic system.

A sluggish lymphatic system can cause enlarged lymph nodes or glands. This situation is common among sedentary people because unlike your bloodstream, which has the heart to pump blood through your veins, your lymphatic system does not have a pump. The only way to increase the lymphatic flow is with lymphatic massage or exercise, especially jumping on a mini-trampoline. Additionally, the use of herbs, such as red clover supports the lymphatic system in filtering toxins from the body.

Cleansing helps every part of your body heal. More importantly, cleansing helps you to shift gears and go from an unhealthy to healthy lifestyle. Cleansing can be the motivational catalyst for other healthier changes in your life. Many people experience some type of greater clarity and even spiritual awareness. You may notice that you are more positive, and feel more energy to get things done. Cleansing improves creativity, and enhances health, beauty and vitality. Skin problems commonly clear up as the liver gets cleansed.

So many of my clients do extremely well in changing their diet, but it may not be enough. Often they reach a plateau if they still can't get off their high-blood pressure medications or lose that last ten pounds. **Cleansing can be the missing piece in both situations.** Even nutritional deficiencies can continue until the digestive system is cleansed. Cleansing is clearly an incredible preventative for many conditions.

Cleansing is also a time when we can get away from the stress of life and turn our thoughts inward where we can get renewed again. Isn't it funny how we take vacations from work to relax and gain a new perspective on life, but we rarely take a break from food? (How can we; it's everywhere!)

Professional cleanses include fiber and certain foods or herbs. In this chapter, we'll look at the many, many benefits of fiber, whole fruits and vegetables and how they will help you to burn fat, lower cholesterol, and achieve great health.

Types of Fiber

Americans suffer from many digestive complaints including colitis, chronic constipation diarrhea, irritable bowel syndrome, Crohn's disease, diverticulitis, hemorrhoids, lack of energy, gas and bloating, varicose veins, kidney problems and gallbladder conditions which are all created by a low-fiber diet. Did you know that increasing the fiber in your diet can help tremendously with most of these problems?

Dietary fiber is a general term we use to describe the non-digestible parts of plant foods. Different fibers have specific effects on your digestion. **The two main types of fiber are water-soluble and non-soluble fiber.**

Water-soluble fiber can dissolve in water and it forms a gel in the gastrointestinal tract by absorbing water and swelling to as much as 10 times its weight. Wow!

Water-soluble fiber sources are found mostly in fruits, vegetables and grains such as oat bran; psyllium seeds, flaxseed, apples, strawberries, squash, cauliflower, broccoli, corn, barley, oatmeal, dried beans (i.e., kidney, navy, split peas, black eyed peas, pinto beans, great northern beans and lentils), baked potatoes and figs. Here are some of the benefits of the water-soluble fiber, psyllium, that is used in the cleanse I recommend in chapter 7.

Benefits of Psyllium

1. It helps to remove fat from the colon wall, so it's good for weight loss. It gives a feeling of fullness which helps keep the appetite normal, and again helps with weight loss.

2. It helps to remove toxic waste from all body systems.

3. It can help lower your blood pressure.

4. It can help protect against heart disease by lowering your level of bad (LDL) cholesterol.

5. It can also help lower blood fats (triglycerides).

6. It can help decrease blood sugar levels by slowing down the absorption of glucose in the intestines. (Blood sugar problems, such as hypoglycemia and diabetes, are related to an inadequate fiber intake.)

Psyllium provides additional fiber to the diet and offers digestive system support when used in a cleansing program. (Be sure to read labels. Many sources of psyllium that you can purchase over-the-counter contain additives, red dyes and artificial sweeteners which are not recommended. I use the Standard Process® product, Gastro-Fiber® as a great source of psyllium in my office.)

Benefits of Non-Soluble Fiber

Non-soluble fibers basically provide roughage because they don't break down during digestion. These are found in wheat bran, whole grain breads and cereals, and some fruits including dates, prunes, peas and lima beans. Wheat bran isn't recommended since it can cause irritation of the colon.

Non-soluble fiber absorbs water and makes the stool larger, softer and easier to pass. It requires plenty of water in the system. This fiber speeds the time it takes food to go through the digestive system, which makes for more complete elimination. So it's an excellent means of controlling constipation, diverticulosis, diarrhea and even preventing hemorrhoids.

There are more than 85,000 colon cancer cases in the United States each year. Yet colon cancer is almost nonexistent in people who eat a high fiber diet. The American Cancer Society recommends that people eat more fiber and less fat as protection against colon cancer. Non-soluble fiber won't cause a lowering of blood fat levels, but it will help in the protection against colon cancer because the fiber collects carcinogens and binds them so they can be removed from the body.

When you start to use fiber in your diet, you should start out small and increase your fiber gradually. (See pages 85-86 about Gastro-Fiber®.) Anyone with any kind of digestive disease should see their doctor before adding a large amount of fiber.

Why Eat Your Veggies?

People have told us for years to eat more fruits and vegetables saying that they are "good for you." But have you ever wondered **how** good they are for us? Or why?

Most of us eat salads for lunch only on occasion. We'll have a side order of cabbage slaw with a burger or a carrot salad at the deli. And the average teenager's idea of veggies is French fries!

General Benefits of Vegetables

Generally speaking your body's natural cleansing system vitally depends on foods. For example, the liver requires foods, such as cabbage, for detoxification. What does that mean to you? **Weight loss! Lower cholesterol! More energy!** The simple, natural fruits and vegetables that surround us are incredible health-supporting foods!

Antioxidants from fruits protect the cell membranes from damaging free radicals generated during the process of detoxification. The kidneys need vitamins, magnesium and potassium for proper excretion. Your intestines require the B complex, fiber and the friendly bacteria for proper function.

Certain vegetables have phytochemicals which can increase our immunity against heart disease, and help lower cholesterol. They have been proven to reduce the incidence of breast, prostate and colon cancers. Broccoli, cauliflower and cabbage, for example, have phytochemical compounds that boost the production of anti-cancer enzymes within hours after they are eaten.

Vegetables and fruits with the deepest colors, like red, orange and green yield the highest antioxidant protection. Lutein, found in kale and broccoli, can protect the macula of the eye and a deficiency of lutein has been linked with macular degeneration.

Lycopene is a carotenoid like beta carotene which is also a powerful antioxidant against cancers and is found in foods like tomatoes, red grapefruit, red peppers and watermelon.

Greens and green foods are high in chlorophyll. Chlorophyll is a substance very similar to our own blood, and is vital for good health. In fact, chlorophyll has nearly an identical molecular structure as our own blood—that means these green foods really nourish our blood.

One of the most important elements of chlorophyll is its affect as a cancer fighter, anti-tumor and anti-viral.

Other foods which are high in chlorophyll include the green leaves from foods such as spinach, collard greens and beet greens. Barley grass, alfalfa and wheat grass are also great green foods. They are also high in iron, magnesium, calcium, manganese, vitamin C, potassium, vitamin A and some of the essential fatty acids. The darker the color, the higher the level of nutrients.

Liver Supporting Foods

According to Dr. Michael Dobbins, certain foods have an incredibly successful effect on the detoxification of the liver. Here are some of the foods that assist in the various parts of Phase 2 detoxification. In other words, these foods help your liver to break down and eliminate toxins and excess fat.

• **Sulfation:** egg yolks, red peppers, garlic, onions, broccoli, brussels sprouts

• **Glutathione conjugation:** asparagus, cabbage, broccoli, brussels sprouts

• **Glucuronidation:** sulphur containing foods as in sulfation.

• **Methylation:** choline, betaine, folic acid, B12.

In chapter 7, I'll present two detoxification or internal cleansing therapies which involve eating foods such as these.

Cruciferous vegetables such as broccoli, cauliflower, cabbage, kale and brussels sprouts all contain phytonutrients such as indole-3-carbinol, which help the liver to detoxify drugs and chemicals. They are also high in antioxidants.

Great Vegetables for Great Health

I've always been motivated to try certain foods when I knew their health benefits. Below are wonderful health-promoting vegetables you'll want to incorporate in your daily meals.

Asparagus: Asparagus is high in chlorophyll and vitamin A, and is also helpful for the kidneys.

Bell pepper, red and green: Rich in vitamin C, peppers help fight off colds, asthma, bronchitis, atherosclerosis and cancer.

Beets: Beets are high in calcium and potassium. Beets are nourishing to the liver and gallbladder by improving bile flow and digestion.

Broccoli: Broccoli is full of fiber, beta carotene and vitamin C. It's also high in bone-building calcium and boron. Broccoli is one of the best anti-cancer vegetables, high in sulforaphane, a powerful antioxidant.

Brussels Sprouts: Brussels sprouts are high in vitamin C, low in sodium, high in potassium and fiber. They are known to inhibit cancer, especially cancer of the colon and stomach.

Cabbage: Cabbage is low in calories, high in fiber, high in vitamin C, and is a cancer-preventing food. Cabbage is said to prevent ulcers and kill bacteria and viruses. The juice stimulates the immune system, and cabbage assists in detoxing the liver.

Carrots: Carrots have been shown to cut the risk of lung cancer, and reduce the blood fats that cause heart attacks and strokes. Carrots are an excellent source of beta carotene, a powerful antioxidant, which is immune boosting and infection fighting. Carrots also help reduce the odds of degenerative eye diseases and are good for healthy skin and teeth.

Cauliflower: Cauliflower is also low in calories, fat and sodium, and high in vitamin C, potassium and is a good source of fiber. Cauliflower helps reduce the risk of cancer, particularly colon, stomach and breast cancer.

Celery: Celery helps lower blood pressure and is good for the heart. Celery also contains anti-cancer compounds and has a calming effect on the nervous system. Celery is good for water retention, weight-loss and cancer.

Cucumbers: Cucumbers aid digestion, cleanse the bowels, and are helpful for breaking up cholesterol deposits. Cucumbers help to promote healthy skin.

Garlic: Garlic contains substances that help lower blood pressure, reduce cholesterol, and hinder the formation of blood clots. Garlic boosts the immune system and acts as a natural antibiotic.

Kale: Kale is high in anti-cancer chemicals, beta carotene and vitamin C which reduces the harmful affects of LDL, and is an easily assimilated source of calcium.

Leeks: A long onion which looks like a large green onion. It's a blood purifier and aid for the liver.

Mushrooms: Mushrooms such as Reishi and Shitake are said to help prevent and treat cancer, viral disease and high-blood cholesterol.

Mustard Greens: Mustard greens act as a decongestant and help break up mucus in air passages. They contain high amounts of calcium, iron, vitamin A and niacin.

Onions: Onions thin the blood, help lower cholesterol, help to prevent strokes and boost HDL, the good cholesterol.

Parsley: Parsley helps the kidneys, bladder, prostate and urinary tract disorders.

Peas: Peas are a good source of cholesterol-lowering soluble fiber. Peas are known to prevent cancer because of carotene and vitamin C.

Pumpkin: Pumpkins are high in beta carotene which has been known to help in cancer, heart attacks and cataracts.

Radishes: Radishes are said to promote digestion, remove mucus, and soothe headaches. Radishes contain vitamins A, B and C.

Spinach: Spinach is high in vitamin A (beta carotene) for eye health, calcium, B vitamins and vitamin E.

Squash: Squash is high in beta carotene, and is said to lower the risk of cancer, particularly lung cancer. Squash helps heal inflammation, relieve pain and soothe the stomach.

Sweet potatoes: (Yams) Sweet Potatoes are high in beta carotene and linked to preventing heart disease.

Great Fruits for Great Health

Without the protection of antioxidants, more free radical damage can occur during detoxification. So antioxidants are vital! Antioxidants are commonly found in fresh raw fruits such as apples, pears, citrus and kiwi fruit and vegetables such as carrots, celery, beets, and green foods.

Apples: Apples can lower blood cholesterol, blood pressure and the risk for cancer. High in soluble fiber, they help prevent sharp mood swings or stabilize blood-sugar levels; they contain a natural appetite suppressant, and are extremely high in potassium.

Avocados: Avocados are good for lowering cholesterol; they benefit circulation. Avocados are high in potassium.

Bananas: Bananas soothe the stomach, prevent and heal ulcers, and help lower cholesterol because of their high amounts of soluble fiber. Bananas help guard against a potassium deficiency.

Berries: Berries contain an antiviral agent and are helpful for urinary tract infections, especially cranberries and blueberries. Berries are high in insoluble fiber and potassium which helps control blood pressure.

Cherries: Cherries are high in potassium and help prevent tooth decay.

Cranberries: Cranberries contain strong antibiotic properties and are known to help fight bladder infections (real unsweetened cranberry juice).

Grapes: Grapes are a good source of boron, and help ward off osteoporosis. Red grapes help prevent artery damage and heart attacks, and lower blood pressure.

Kiwifruit: Kiwifruit is packed with nutrients, especially vitamin C and fiber.

Lemon: Lemons regenerate the liver, strengthen the stomach acids and salivary enzymes, and help the pancreas, thyroid and adrenal glands.

Mango: Mangos help lower blood pressure, and are high in beta carotene and vitamin C.

Melon: Melons contain the antioxidant beta carotene and are high in fiber, potassium and vitamin C.

Oranges: Oranges are high in vitamin C and folic acid which fight birth defects. Oranges are rich in antioxidants and beta carotene and may ward off asthma, bronchitis and breast cancer.

Papaya: Papayas are high in vitamins C and A; and are helpful in digestive problems.

Peaches: High in Vitamin A, peaches are an alkaline fruit with a laxative effect.

Pears: Pears are a great source of fiber, and help reduce the risk of developing polyps of the colon.

Pineapple: Pineapples contain bromelain, an anti-inflammatory. Pineapple is said to aid digestion, dissolve blood clots and help prevent osteoporosis.

So now you might be wondering how to incorporate these wonderful foods into your daily meals or cleanse.

Let's go on to part 5, which tells you how to design your life for health through internal cleansing.

PART FIVE

How To Design Your Life for Health

Chapter Seven

How Do I Cleanse?

Recently I was speaking to a group of women who asked me questions about how to feel better, stay young and lose weight. I told them that there was a simple answer that could do all of these and more: Cleanse! I could see the expression on their faces change as they realized what this might mean. Perhaps they were remembering their last experience just trying to go without **one** meal, much less many meals!

While cleansing isn't the easiest thing in the world, I've found a cleanse that is both livable and effective. Backed by clinical research, this plan can be followed from seven to twenty-one days with simple, natural foods. It's designed so any person can follow it while still engaging in their normal activities.

Of course, there are questions before the cleanse as well, the main one being: "How close to a toilet will I have to be?"

Who Should Cleanse?

Nearly everyone can benefit from cleansing, especially anyone who feels just lousy! Several female clients, following a cleanse, noticed a reduction in the severity of PMS symptoms, and symptoms related to menopause and pre-menopause.

Cleansing is ideal for people who complain of fatigue and are overweight. Many people trying to lose weight aren't just overweight; they're also toxic.

However, there are several conditions that require medical supervision. Do not cleanse without checking with your primary health care provider if you fall into any of the following categories:

- You are pregnant or lactating
- You take prescription medications
- You have a long-term illness
- You have a genetic disease
- You have severe liver problems
- You have an autoimmune disorder

Finding Time to Cleanse

Most people can't take time off from their busy schedules to fast. But nearly everyone can cleanse if they use whole foods which help them maintain normal blood-sugar levels. That's why I prefer the newer, more effective ways to cleanse.

New and Updated Cleansing

Many people imagine that the best way to cleanse is by water fasting. However, clinical research now shows that prolonged water fasting may **suppress** detoxification rather than enhance it, and weaken muscles and organs because of protein loss and reduced metabolic activity.

In the last thirty years, I've tried dozens of ways to fast including a juice fast. I remember being very tired, discouraged, and that I would gain back the weight I would lose. I've found both personally and professionally, that just drinking juices causes an unstable blood-sugar level, fatigue, and high-insulin levels. This can lead to further stress on the glands as well as eventual weight gain.

There are literally thousands of diets for health and weight loss. The goal for each is to:

1. Lower insulin levels.
2. Eliminate junk foods.
3. Insure liver detoxification with food, protein, fiber and herbs.
4. Assist the liver in pumping out excess fat.

A far more effective way to achieve these goals is through the use of a protein supplement, fiber and specific nutrition for the liver, colon and other organs of elimination.

You Need Protein!

Protein nourishes the body, feeding the natural detoxification activity. By giving the body high quality protein, vegetables, fruits and essential fat, the body gets what it needs to prevent muscle breakdown and energy depletion.

According to a study in the *Annual Review of Nutrition,* the Cytochrome P450 detoxification process family of enzymes depends on adequate dietary protein. Protein is so important that protein deficiency states can result in **decreased** liver detoxification of many drugs.[38] Fasting, which involves protein restriction can result in lowered detoxification ability, and according to *Archives of Environmental Health,* can increase the toxic effect of some chemicals.[39]

Refined carbohydrates also reduce the ability of the P450 enzymes to work effectively.[40] According to research from the *British Journal of Clinical Pharmacology*, a diet that is well balanced in protein and lower in total carbohydrates may provide the optimal activation of Cytochrome P450 enzymes.[41] Fats are valuable because they provide an additional energy source.

Various Approaches to Cleansing

Dr. Michael Dobbins, after studying the liver and discovering nutrients that support the liver, designed a liver detoxification supplement program that incorporates dried, whole-food supplements which contain these specific cleansing foods. I list these on the next page. (To obtain the supplements that he recommends, see your natural health care professional or clinical nutritionist to order any of the products from Standard Process® or MediHerb®.)

You can follow his liver cleanse while eating plenty of vegetables, lean meat or fish. You'll see a list of foods to eliminate, including all processed and refined foods, especially sugar. **The number in parenthesis is the recommended daily dosage of the supplements he lists.**

Dr. Dobbin's Liver Detox Protocol

- Hepatrophin PMG® (3) (For liver disease or degeneration)
- St. John's Wort-IMT™ (3) (Doubles the action of Phase 1 and 2)
- LivCo® (3) (Helps support Phase 1 and 2 detoxification)
- A-F Betafood® (6) (Beet roots, leaves, carrots and other nutrients which support a healthy liver function.)
- Garlic (*Organically Grown*) (2) (Assists in Phase 2 detoxification glucuronidation)
- Cruciferous Complete™ (6) (formerly called Phytolyn)
- SP Green Food™ (6) (natural antioxidants)
- Spanish Black Radish (6) (natural source of MSM)
- Cholacol 2® (6-12) (Assists in moving the bowels)

Dr. Dobbins recommends the above-listed supplements for one to three weeks. He suggests that if the cleansing process is too aggressive, take out or reduce the St. John's Wort-IMT™ or LivCo®. If you have more gas than usual, don't worry—it's working! Be sure to drink plenty of water and get moderate exercise. The goal of any cleanse is to both lower insulin levels, and cleanse the liver.

Eliminate These Foods and Beverages

- White sugar and snack foods made with white sugar
- White flour and foods made with white flour
- Fast food and fried foods
- Processed and refined foods
- Hydrogenated and partially hydrogenated fats (margarine and Crisco)
- Processed vegetable oils
- Preserved meats such as: bacon, salami, hog dogs and sausage
- Caffeine, alcohol, soft drinks, diet colas & carbonated drinks
- Chocolate and chocolate-based products, dyed teas
- French fries, corn products, potatoes, and potato chips

(For more information, you can contact Dr. Dobbins through his web page at www.dobbins.org.)

Another tip: Be sure to have lots of toilet paper on hand. I'd say about 24 rolls should do it!

A Clinical Cleanse

I have finally found and have used a cleanse personally and professionally more than a year, with continual excellent results. It's called the **Standard Process purification (Cleansing) program.**[42] It includes a fiber called Gastro-Fiber®, a liver cleanse called SP Cleanse®, a whey protein supplement shake called SP Complete™, and organically grown, dried green foods called SP Green Food™.

SP Complete™

We need protein to raise the body's metabolism for fat loss, to insure proper cleansing in the liver, and to stimulate the pancreas to produce glucagon. Without protein, the body loses muscle tissue. Whey-based protein drinks are easy to use, support immune function, and protect lean body mass. Whey protein is extremely soluble with a higher Biological Value than eggs. For example, whey protein has 104 BV, beef has 80 BV, and eggs have 100 BV.

SP Complete is far superior to most commercial whey-protein drinks since it's non-denatured and therefore doesn't cause gastrointestinal problems as other whey protein drinks may. SP Complete provides essential vitamins and minerals to the body during detoxification or for a morning shake or meal replacement.

Here are a few of the components of SP Complete:
- **Ginkgo biloba and grape seed:** excellent antioxidants
- **Carrot powder:** excellent source of the vitamin A complex
- **Alfalfa powder:** cleanses the lymph glands, and a great antioxidant
- **Barley grass juice:** cleanses lymph glands and a great antimicrobial
- **Brussels sprouts and kale powder:** excellent liver food

Gastro-Fiber®

Fiber acts like a broom, sweeping the colon lining. Fiber is vital for cleansing because if not enough fiber is present, the toxins are reabsorbed in the body. (See earlier chapter on the benefits of soluble and insoluble fiber on pages 60 and 72-74.)

Gastro-Fiber is a completely vegetarian product formulated specifically to provide additional fiber to any healthy diet. Gastro-Fiber **contains soluble and insoluble fibers including: Psyllium husk powder, collinsonia root powder, apple pectin, fennel and fenugreek plus their synergistic co-factors.**

SP Cleanse®

Many different plants and herbs contain ingredients that enhance the body's ability to efficiently remove both metabolic and environmental toxins. SP Cleanse is a combination of over 20 of these whole foods and botanicals, rich in phytonutrients, that help the body cleanse itself from the inside out-naturally.

Here are a few of the components of SP Cleanse:

• **Juniper berry powder:** diuretic and urinary antiseptic

• **Red clover flower:** cleanses blood and supports immune system

• **Collinsonia root:** increases strength of peristalsis

• **Burdock root powder:** cleanses lymph, and is an antimicrobial

• **Barley grass powder:** source of chlorophyll, a liver cleansing agent

Together these nutrients help support bile production, pull fat from the liver, and break down fat and toxins.

SP Green Food™

Most people don't like or eat green vegetables, but our liver depends on green foods for cleansing! SP Green Food™ contains: **Buckwheat juice powder, barley grass juice powder, brussels sprouts powder, kale powder, and alfalfa sprout powder.**

All of these foods are high in chlorophyll, minerals, vitamins A, C, E, K, and B12, and amino acids, which all support internal cleansing.

How Do I Cleanse?

There are two plans presented on the next pages:* **Garden Variety** (Optimal Intensity Program) for the person who wants to lose weight, and **Wholesome Medley** (Modified Program) for the person who can't afford to lose weight. Both plans follow the Standard Process purification program which includes the shake mix, fruits and vegetables. The second program adds some animal protein and some brown rice which makes the cleanse easier.

I usually wait 1-3 months before I recommend this cleanse, but some of my clients are ready on the first appointment! If my clients have never cleansed, I have them try it for a day or so, or do it once a week, for a few months. They are generally surprised at how easy it is to follow, and they often want to follow it longer. These programs are designed for 3 weeks. I've even had clients follow it for 6 or more weeks. Some clients like to do this cleanse once or twice a year.

Reprinted with Permission from the Standard Process purification program.

1. Garden Variety: Optimal Intensity Program

Food Intake: Weeks 1-3

For the first three weeks, consume only the items listed here in addition to your supplementation. Use organic fruits and vegetables if available.

- **Unlimited fresh vegetables**

o Collard greens*	Radishes
o Dandelion greens	Kale*
o Mixed greens	Broccoli*
o Mustard greens	Swiss chard
o Red, yellow, and green peppers	Brussels sprouts
o Onions*	Asparagus*
o Mushrooms	Cabbage*
o Spinach	Red beets (Beets may be steamed for 20-30 minutes or until soft. Use the beet greens in your salad after washing.
o Carrots	Celery
o Cucumbers	

May be steamed for four minutes*

- **Salads with unlimited fresh vegetables**
    - o *Salad dressings (including lemon juice) are not permissible*
    - o *Nuts, seeds, and beans (including green beans) are not permissible*
- **Fruit—eat twice as many vegetables as compared to fruit (1 serving = 1 cup)**
    - o Examples include but not limited to:

·Apples	Berries
·Oranges	Melons
·Bananas	Tomatoes
·Grapes	

    - o *Avocadoes and lemons are not permissible*

- **Spring water (at least 8 glasses per day)**

Refrain from consuming anything not listed.

Supplementation: Garden Variety

SP Complete™ and Gastro-Fiber® are recommended throughout the Garden Variety program, SP Cleanse® is recommended for week one only, and SP Green Food™ is recommended for weeks two and three.

Week One
* 2-3 SP Complete shakes per day
* 7 SP Cleanse, 3 times daily
* 3 Gastro-Fiber capsules, 3 times daily

Weeks Two & Three
* 2-3 SP Complete shakes per day
* 3 Gastro-Fiber capsules, 3 times daily
* 5 SP Green Food capsules, 2 times daily

Please note that supplements should be taken with an SP Complete shake or water, but not with food. The supplements may also be taken right before bed.

Exercise

Walk at least 4 times per week for 30-45 minutes. This gets your lymphatic system moving. Put strenuous exercise on hold during the three-week period. Consult your health care professional if you are currently on an exercise program that you would like to maintain throughout the cleanse.

SP Complete Supplement Shake Recipe

2 rounded tablespoons (scoops) of SP Complete
1-2 cups of water (increase for desired consistency)
1/2 cup of your favorite fruit (examples include berries, bananas, peaches, apples, or cherries)
2 teaspoons high-quality oil such as flaxseed oil

Directions:

Blend all ingredients together. Wait a few minutes and then add additional water and/or fruit until you achieve the desired consistency and flavor. This recipe could be doubled or tripled to make a large enough batch to last you 1-2 days, but make sure to keep it refrigerated, and remix it as needed before pouring. *Recipe may be varied according to personal taste.*

My note about the shake. To get the best results, skip the milk, soy milk, rice milk, and so on, and just use water. But whey protein doesn't taste very good, so to get it to taste good, you **must** add the fruit. At the end of this chapter, I'll explain why this fruit is really vital. Whatever you do, don't add sugar! (I like using stevia, a naturally sweet herb.)

2. Wholesome Medley: Modified Program

Food Intake: Weeks 1-3

For the first three weeks, consume only the items listed here in addition to your supplementation. Use organic fruits and vegetables if available.

- **3-4 oz. of unseasoned meat, fish, or poultry twice daily** *(simply prepared - broiling, baking, etc.)*
- **Unlimited fresh vegetables**

o Collard greens*	Radishes
o Dandelion greens	Kale*
o Mixed greens	Broccoli*
o Mustard greens	Swiss chard
o Red, yellow, and green peppers	Brussels sprouts
o Onions*	Asparagus*
o Mushrooms	Cabbage*
o Spinach	Red beets (Beets may be steamed for 20-30 minutes or until soft. Use the beet greens in your salad after washing.
o Carrots	Celery
o Cucumbers	

  May be steamed for four minutes*
- **Salads with unlimited fresh vegetables**
  - *Salad dressings (including lemon juice) are not permissible*
  - *Nuts, seeds, and beans (including green beans) are not permissible*
- **Fruit—eat twice as many vegetables as compared to fruit (1 serving = 1 cup)**

o   Examples include but not limited to:

· Apples	Berries
· Oranges	Melons
· Bananas	Tomatoes
· Grapes	

o   *Avocadoes and lemons are not permissible*

- **2 servings of brown or wild rice (not instant) per day (1 serving = 1 cup)**

- **Spring water (at least 8 glasses per day)**
  Refrain from consuming anything not listed.

Supplementation: Wholesome Medley

SP Complete™ and Gastro-Fiber® are recommended throughout the entire program, SP Cleanse® is recommended for week one only, and SP Green Food™ is recommended for weeks two and three.

Week One
- 2-3 SP Complete shakes per day
- 7 SP Cleanse capsules, 3 times daily
- 3 Gastro-Fiber capsules, 3 times daily

Weeks Two & Three
- 2-3 SP Complete shakes per day
- 3 Gastro-Fiber capsules, 3 times daily
- 5 SP Green Food capsules, 2 times daily

Please note that supplements should be taken with an SP Complete shake or water, but not with food. The supplements may also be taken right before bed.

Exercise

Walk at least 4 times per week for 30-45 minutes. This gets your lymphatic system moving. Put strenuous exercise on hold during the three-week period. Consult your health care professional if you are currently on an exercise program that you would like to maintain throughout the cleanse.

Please, don't give up in the middle of the cleanse and have some ice cream or coffee! It's better not to cleanse than to take these toxic substances while you are cleansing because you have opened the pathways of detoxification, and you would just do further harm with these stimulants. So you really have to get mentally prepared ahead of time for cleansing.

Don't Think You Can Do It?

Okay, I'm sure there are some of you who would like to try something like this, but perhaps you have tried in the past and only lasted a day or so. What can you do?

At the time of this writing, all of my assistants in the office have done, or are doing the cleanse. They have found time in their schedules in which to do the cleanse. Some of them are doing great. One of them sometimes has trouble following a cleanse such as this. I asked Anne how she handled it. Here's her answer:

"This time, I asked my husband to get involved. To my surprise, he said, 'Yes!' Now, we are both following the cleanse and he's helping me so much. When I get in a place where I want to cheat and go off the cleanse, Wayne keeps me motivated. Now I don't have to cook different meals for each of us. It's much easier this way! And he's doing great. He just said yesterday that he couldn't believe how great grapefruit juice tasted! I don't even want a coke, and when I did taste one recently, it tasted awful! Lorrie explained that we're healing our taste buds as well as our bodies and that foods will taste better now, and junk foods will not taste as good."

After the Initial Three Weeks

So you might be wondering how to continue after your cleanse. After two weeks, you'll want to check with your health professional for length of time on the cleanse, because it will vary for each person. In the next chapter, I explain how to begin eating normal foods. I've lost weight and kept it off through a combination of cleansing and following a low-carbohydrate eating plan. Dr. Michael Dobbins lost 120 pounds following a low-carbohydrate diet. In the next chapter, I'll give a typical day of menus from both myself and Dr. Dobbins.

I interviewed Dr. Dobbins regarding his program and his successful weight loss. Here is his encouraging testimony.

Dr. Dobbin's Testimony

"My life, it seemed, had been one long battle with weight. When I was a child my pants were always "husky" size—made me think I was a new breed of dog! I was a sugar-addict if there ever was one. I started every day with not less than one-half cup of sugar on top of some sort of cereal. I remember lunchtime being little more than a "challenge time" to obtain and eat as many of the "desserts" available as possible. Before long I weighed 120 pounds more than I should, and I knew it. But what we know and what we do are certainly not always related! Once I learned the incredible impact of carbohydrates on my weight and over-all health I began the process of permanently changing the way I eat. I keep my carbohydrates very low and concentrate on good protein, good fats and on the good, liver supporting vegetables discussed in this book. The 120 pounds is history and I play racquetball better and longer now than I did 20 years ago! The principles of sound eating are NOT difficult to follow—once you really, really decide to do it."

By the way, Dr. Dobbins was the one who came up with the idea and the one who primarily tested the high-protein, carbohydrate controlled Standard Process Cocoa Cherry StandardBar.® These bars are convenient and taste great, yet they provide a balance of important nutrients your body needs from whole-food sources. Here are some benefits that make these bars a great part of any weight-loss plan:

- They are easy to pack in your lunch or take for snacks
- They contain 17 grams of protein and a net carbohydrate count of 5 grams
- They taste great and help curb sugar cravings
- They contain carbohydrates of the beneficial complex form as opposed to simple sugar
- They satisfy vegetarian diet requirements
- They enhance energy through increased protein content

What About Eating Fruit?

If you've ever followed a high-protein diet, the first thing you might wonder is why there is so much fruit in this plan. People often ask me about the glycemic index of certain fruits as related to weight loss. In fact, I've seen glycemic index charts that would make refined sugar lower than a banana! Obviously, we are concerned with the nutrition in foods in a case such as this. The banana is a better choice than the refined sugar!

To assist in "counting" carbohydrates, I got permission from Dr. Bond to reprint a chart from one of his seminars which compares the amount of carbohydrates in fruits and vegetables to other carbohydrates.

Notice on the charts on the next page that vegetables are really low, fruits are somewhat higher, but starches such as bagels and spaghetti are very high! These are the foods that raise your insulin levels. By using protein, fruits and vegetables, you can both lower your insulin levels and also maintain normal blood-sugar levels while assisting the liver to burn fat.

However, as I mentioned earlier in this book, if you don't lose weight following this cleanse, don't give up! You may be insulin resistant, and like my client Mary, you may want to follow a low-carbohydrate eating plan, without fruits, before you follow this plan. After your insulin levels come down, it will be easier. I would also recommend that you take Gymnema 4g from MediHerb® for that purpose as well. Also, you may be a person who has to follow it once, twice, or several times before all the weight comes off. I've had a client once who worked with me for six months before she lost any significant weight. Following that sixth month, she lost 70 pounds! Don't give up, and give it enough time!

Comparison of Carbohydrates With Vegetables

Vegetable	Carb Gms.	Other Carbohydrates	Carb Gms.
Broccoli (1 cup)	6 grams	Spaghetti (1 cup)	37 grams
Pepper (1 medium)	6 grams	Bagel (1 medium)	64 grams
Kale (1 cup)	8 grams	Brown rice (1 cup)	46 grams
Swiss Chard (1 cup)	7 grams	Grape Nut Raisin Cereal™ (1 cup)	96 grams
Tomato (1 medium)	8 grams	Navy, Kidney, Red Beans (1 cup)	126 grams
Beets (1 cup)	12 grams	Almonds (1 cup)	34 grams

Comparison of Carbohydrates With Fruits

Fruit	Carb Gms.	Other Carbohydrates	Carb Gms.
Berries (1 cup)	20 grams	Spaghetti (1 cup)	37 grams
Apple (1 medium)	23 grams	Bagel (1 medium)	64 grams
Banana (1 medium)	20 grams	Brown rice (1 cup)	46 grams
Strawberries (1 cup)	10 grams	Grape Nut Raisin Cereal™ (1 cup)	96 grams
Orange (1 medium)	17 grams	Navy, Kidney, Red Beans (1 cup)	126 grams
Pineapple (1 thick slice)	10 grams	Almonds (1 cup)	34 grams

In summary, eating a lean protein (whey), lots of vegetables, and a few fruits is a terrific balance for internal cleansing, weight loss and energy.

Let's move on to learn what to expect during cleansing and how to design your life after cleansing.

Chapter Eight

What Should I Expect During & After Cleansing?

Cleansing is quite a challenge for most people, especially if they are used to eating several fast food meals a day. When you actually begin to allow the body to cleanse, the process of eliminating these toxins can be somewhat uncomfortable!

So often when people begin to change their diet and/or follow a cleansing program, their body finally has the nutrients and opportunity to begin releasing chemicals and toxins. A cold, for example, is the body's process of detoxification. The runny nose is a sign of increased mucus as the body eliminates virus particles. Yet, we are so used to treating the symptoms or suppressing the symptoms with drugs.

According to Dr. Joel Fuhrman in *Fasting and Eating for Health*, a fever aids the body's immune defenses, activates the white blood cells, and induces interferon secretion (a substance that helps the immune system become active). He says that by drugging away our symptoms, people keep themselves sick longer and can turn a minor disease into a major one![43]

It's helpful to discuss some possible discomforts of cleansing (especially if you want to remain friends!). Remember, these symptoms are generated by your body during the cleansing process and are not any cause for alarm.

As the body discards toxins, (from coffee, for example), it removes them from the tissue and transports them through the bloodstream, which we experience as pain—a headache! We want to stop the pain by taking some Aspirin, but that's the **last** thing we should do.

So I encourage my clients to properly **prepare** for cleansing by eating more fruits and vegetables and eliminating processed foods **before** they cleanse. The better you eat before the cleanse, the easier the cleanse will be!

What about coffee and/or caffeine? **Give it up before you cleanse!** There are many points of view on this, but I take the gentler approach. I recommend that you cut your caffeine consumption in half the first week. That means if you drank twenty cups of coffee per day (yes, there are some people who do!), then cut it in half the first week, or down to 10 cups. If you drank three cups, cut down to 1 1/2 cups the first week. Keep cutting it in half until you are off caffeine. Then you can cleanse. (But, if you are the go-getter type, then just cold-turkey it! But remember, don't take Aspirin!)

Most people need caffeine because they are tired! In the meantime, take supplements according to your health professional's recommendation to increase your energy and support your thyroid or adrenal glands in the process. (You might want my book, *Why Am I So Grumpy, Dopey and Sleepy?* about energy listed on the back page of this book.)

What Else Happens During a Cleanse?

Here is a good explanation of why you might locate the toilets nearest you! (Taken from the SP Purification brochure[44]):

> For some people going through the purification program, the frequency and quantity of urination increases. This is a normal reaction as the body begins to burn fat and natural insulin levels drop. This will level out after a few days. Some people also notice an increase in the quantity of bowel movements. This again is normal. Most people today have forgotten what a complete bowel movement entails. In rare instances, there may be a day or two of the head feeling tight, generalized aches, itchy skin, or fatigue. These are normal occurrences as the body detoxifies and will pass after a day or two.

According to Dr. Donna Smith, "Remember that the greatest source for all pain in the body is all of the toxins stored in your cells and tissues. Toxins include chemicals, germs, etc. So if pain is caused by toxins in the body, it makes sense that you can feel pain or discomfort when these toxins and germs are moving through the body on their way out! However, the signs of pain and discomfort as a result of cleansing **are not lasting or harmful,** unlike those associated with disease that eventually occur when toxins stay in the body for years."

I've observed in the last 20 years of supervising cleanses, that side effects of cleansing can include: Headaches and fatigue, fever, chill, skin eruptions, constipation, diarrhea, nervousness, frequent urination and some symptoms similar to the cold or flu. It's also common to experience bad breath and smelly urine and stools. You'll be glad that this stuff is finally being eliminated!

You may experience some skin eruptions in the cleansing process, which should go away quickly. You may even experience nausea or vomiting. If you do, Phosfood Liquid® is available from Standard Process® to eliminate the sludge trapped in your gallbladder which causes vomiting. Take 10 drops in 1/4 to 1 cup of water as needed.

A Possible Explanation of Healing

Here is a side note that was given to me by Dr. Donna Smith about the order in which your body cleanses.

According to Bernard Jensen, there is an order of healing and this order is often observed in a cleansing program. You may notice signs of healing in the following order: From the head down, from the inside out, and in reverse order from its onset.

In other words, problems in the head clear up before problems with your feet. Problems with vital organs and glands (the heart, adrenals, kidneys, lower stomach, and colon) clear up before skin problems. And if you have suffered for years with first stomachaches, Athlete's foot, poor or short-term memory, and then boils, you may notice your boils clear up first, then your short-term memory is restored, then Athlete's foot clears up, and then your stomach heals.

Getting and Staying Motivated

As a motivational speaker, I would highly suggest that you set a goal. Make it fun; for example, why not have a contest among your family members. The one who loses the most weight gets to go to Hawaii. (Hey, can I go with? I've never been to Hawaii!)

Whatever you do, don't have a bunch of cooking magazines laying around, and try not to watch too much TV. You don't need to watch commercials with ice cream sundaes and foods dripping with cheese or chocolate while you are cleansing! The best thing to do really is to read books about cleansing such as this one! You'll stay motivated if you continue to remind yourself of what you are doing (cleansing) and why you are doing it (for health, weight loss, and energy.)

The more rest, water and sleep you get, the easier the cleanse. Realize that by eliminating these toxins you are preventing many diseases. If you already exercise, continue at a moderate pace.

As always, you will want to discuss serious medical conditions with your health care practitioner. It helps, by the way, to find a natural health care practitioner who also cleanses! If he/she has never cleansed, how can he/she discuss the whole process with you at a personal level?

Upon completion of the three week purification program you will have a different attitude regarding your body and towards food. Once your body is accustomed to eating this way, you'll notice the desire for junk foods is gone, and cravings for certain foods such as sugar and chocolate may disappear. This is good!

Re-Entry Schedule

Following the cleanse is a good time to identify your food allergies, if any. Try eating each of the foods listed on the next page (possible allergens) for three days and see how you feel. Choose one food at a time and eat it for 3 days in a row; then choose another food to test. Repeat this process.

Possible Allergens

- Dairy products
- Eggs
- Peanuts
- Wheat products
- Corn products
- Sugar

If you experience reactions such as headaches, digestive problems, or sinus problems, those foods are allergens to you. The Pulse Test can also help. Take your resting pulse. Then eat one food and check your pulse before and 30 minutes after each food. If your pulse raises ten points or more, you may have an allergy to this food, which causes more toxicity and hinders weight loss. (For more information, see my first book, *Why Can't I Lose Weight?*)

After cleansing, many people continue to drink a shake either as their breakfast or in conjunction with their breakfast. The SP Complete is a wonderful way to obtain a whole variety of essential vital nutrients in an enjoyable, tasty way.

Lunch or dinner could consist of some protein (fish or chicken) and a large salad or steamed vegetables. Eating low-glycemic foods contributes to normal blood-sugar levels.

I asked Dr. Dobbins how he maintains his weight loss. Since he travels extensively, many of his meals are at restaurants. He tries not to eat more than 50 grams of carbohydrates daily. He never eats pasta or bread since it makes him feel bloated. Here is his typical daily menu:

Breakfast:	A low-carb bar (StandardBar®) or 1-2 eggs with a piece of fruit, preferably honeydew, cantaloupe or strawberries, plus a high-fat cheese
Mid-morning:	A piece of fruit or low-carb bar
Lunch:	A Chef salad with blue cheese dressing or Chicken or tuna salad with a side of coleslaw
Mid-afternoon snack:	A low-carb bar, or cheese or handful of nuts
Dinner:	4-5 ounces of meat, fish or chicken

I've also lost weight following a low-carbohydrate diet. I really enjoy the SP purification program and often drink the SP Complete as a meal replacement. Here's my typical day:

Breakfast:	SP Complete shake (as outlined in this book)
	and/or 1-2 eggs with a piece of fruit
Mid-morning:	A piece of fruit or low-carb bar (StandardBar®)
Lunch:	A green salad with chicken or
	SP Complete shake and/or a low-carb bar.
Mid-afternoon snack:	A piece of fruit and/or low-carb bar
Dinner:	4-5 ounces of meat, fish or chicken
	A green salad with lots of vegetables
	2-3 steamed vegetables (I love asparagus!)

The Joy of Cooking Vegetables

So now you've at least read about cleansing and the incredible benefits of eating fruits and vegetables. Perhaps you are ready to try it yourself for a day, or even a week or two. The more you cleanse and eat natural foods, the less you will even want junk foods!

We have become a fast-food nation and natural cooking has become a lost art in this country. As a young woman, I went to Boston and California to study natural food cooking, and I'm glad I did. But good health doesn't require fancy recipes; just whole, natural foods. After cleansing, you will appreciate simple food; especially fresh fruits and vegetables.

In closing, taking care of your body is your privilege as well as your responsibility. Something happens when you realize personally that you are not at the mercy of the latest study, pill or doctor, and that your body wants to, and is designed to heal itself. And you'll feel so victorious because cleansing is definitely a discipline.

If you need additional help in the area of supplements, hormones, weight loss, motivation or energy, you can find a list of my books at the end of this book. (For information on any of the products mentioned in this book, and the web pages of the doctors mentioned in this book, see the Appendix on the next page.)

May God bless you on your journey to health!

How to Find Products and a Natural Health Professional

In writing this book on internal body cleansing or detoxification, one of my goals was to help the readers understand the importance of cleansing and what to expect when doing a cleansing program. The products you will need to do the most effective cleansing program that I have found are available only through natural health professionals who use Standard Process® whole-food supplements, and MediHerb® herbal supplements. The supplements you use in your cleansing program or any health improvement program are the determining factor as to whether your body will be able to cleanse thoroughly, heal itself properly, and achieve your goals, from weight loss to lowering cholesterol.

You wouldn't eat junk food while trying to improve your health, and you certainly wouldn't want to use junk vitamins (synthetic or crystalline extract vitamins), that are sold in most stores or provided through direct mail order vitamin companies. In my book, *Why Do I Need Whole-Food Supplements*, I have explained with clinical research why whole-food vitamin supplements are the only type of supplements that promotes both short- and long-term healing and health. Standard Process Inc. sells whole-food vitamin supplements through natural health professionals.

So when you are ready to do your cleansing program and/or seek professional help to improve any health concern you have, it will be important for you to find a "natural" health professional who can provide the products I have recommended in this book.

Not all doctors, dietitians or nutritionists have been trained in how to evaluate your health and assist you in improving and maintaining health using the methods and products I have recommended in this and other books I have written. In fact, many are still following the outdated Food Pyramid, and ignoring completely the scientifically proven facts that high amounts of carbohydrates are detrimental to our health. Most people vitally need to take supplements in the form of whole-food supplements, and many imbalances in the body can be helped through internal cleansing as described in this book.

The recommendations in my books are based upon years of safe and successful results for myself, personally, and professionally for thousands of clients I have helped since 1997. Every idea and product mentioned in this book is backed by clinical science.

So the type of "natural" health professional you want to assist you in internal body detoxification and health improvement are Naturopathic Doctors (N.D.), Clinical Nutritionists (C.N.), Certified Clinical Nutritionists (C.C.N.), and any doctor (D.C., M.D., D.D., D.O., D.D.S., Ph.D.) or pharmacists who has studied and even completed post-graduate studies in Clinical Nutrition.

Be selective and careful when you choose a professional nutritionist. Make sure they are more interested in you than your money! And inquire about their education. (I would recommend you find a C.N., C.C.N., or C.N.S. All require rigorous training programs, and they require continuing education requirements to maintain a license.)

These "natural" health professionals have been trained in how to nutritionally interpret various types of biochemical tests as well as how to provide other safe and effective methods to evaluate your health status, such as identifying vitamin and mineral deficiencies.

The quickest way to find a natural health professional who can provide whole-food supplements for your cleanse is to contact Standard Process Inc. and ask for the name and number of the nearest natural health professional who uses Standard Process products in their practice.

About Standard Process Products

Standard Process products are only available through "natural" health professionals as listed on the previous page. If you purchase vitamins from a health food store or through the mail, I can't guarantee you the same results as with a clinical product such as Standard Process.

You can call or write Standard Process to locate a health professional in your area:

Standard Process Inc. and MediHerb
1200 West Royal Lee Drive
Palmyra, WI 53156-0904
1-800-848-5061

I'm grateful for the help and knowledge from the following doctors who have contributed greatly to this book.

Dr. Michael Dobbins
1240 High Street
Alameda, CA 94501
510-747-1600
Web address: www.dobbins.org

Dr. Donna Smith, Ph.D., CCN
1911 Tilden Street
Wichita Falls, TX 76309
940-761-4045
Web address: www.womensportsnutrition.com
E-mail: wsnqas@aol.com

Dr. Bruce Bond
26250 Euclid Ave, Suite 509
Euclid, OH 44132
216-289-1114

Dr. Janet Lang
19191 Falzone Road
Wildwood, MO 63038
Web address: www.drjlang.com
E-mail: doctorlang@aol.com

If any of you would like to contact me, my address is listed below. My bio and booklist are at the end of this book.

Lorrie Medford, CN
Life Design Nutrition
9726 E. 42nd St. Suite 231
Tulsa, OK 74146
918-664-4483
918-664-0300 (fax)
Web address: lifedesignnutrition.com
E-mail: Lorrie@lifedesignnutrition.com

Endnotes

1. Dr. John Lee, *Medical Letter,* June, 2001, pp. 1-3.

2. Dr. Royal Lee, "The Special Nutritional Qualities of Natural Foods," 1942, Report #4, p. 43.

3. Paul Stitt, *Fighting the Food Giants,* (Manitowoc, WI: Natural Press), pp. 40-41.

4. Dr. Linda Berry, *Internal Cleansing,* (Roseville, CA: Prima Publishing, 2000), p. 66.

5. Ibid, p. 67.

6. Warren Leon and Caroline Smith DeWaal, *Is Our Food Safe?* (New York, NY: Three Rivers Press), 2002, pp. 83-86.

7. Ibid.p. 87.

8. Ibid, p. 82.

9. Patrick Quillin, Ph.D., *Immunopower* (Tulsa, OK: Nutrition Times, 2000), p. 122.

10. Peter Bennett, N.D., *Seven-Day Detox Miracle,* (Rocklin, CA: Prima, 1999), pp. 28-36.

11. Dr. Bruce Bond, Euclid, OH: *Detoxification/Purification* Seminar, 2003.

12. Lindsey Duncan, "Internal Detoxification" Healthy and Natural Journal, October 1988, p. 2.

13. Lorrie Medford, *Why Can't I Lose Weight?* (Tulsa, OK: LDN Publishing, 1999), pp. 31-33.

14. Dr. Sandra Cabot, *The Healthy Liver and Bowel Book,* (Cobbitty, Australia, 1999), pp. 17-18.

15. *Tulsa World,* Aug 29, 1995, p. 12.

16. Dr. Janet Lang, Lang Nutritional Seminars, Wildwood, MO, *Fibromyalgia and Chronic Fatigue,* 2002.

17. Dr. Michael Murray, *The Encyclopedia of Natural Medicine,* Rocklin, CA: Prima Publishing, p. 520-521.

18. Dr. Michael Murray, *Health Counselor,* Vol. 4, No. 6, p. 32.

19. Dr. Earl Mindell, *Prescription Alternatives* (Los Angeles, CA: Keats Publishing), p. 185.

20. Dr. Michael Murray, *The Encyclopedia of Natural Medicine,* p. 520.

21. Ann Louise Gittleman, *The Fat Flush Plan,* (New York, NY: McGraw Hill, 2002), p. 13.

22. Dr. Jonathan Wright, *Dr. Wright's Guide to Healing With Nutrition,* (New Canaan, CT: Keats Publishing, Inc., 1984), pp. 51-52.

23. Dr. Jon Matsen, *The Mysterious Cause of All Illness,* (Canfield, OH: Fischer Publishing, 1987), pp. 7-9.

24. Ibid.

25. H. Leighton Steward et al., *Sugar Busters!* (New York, NY: The Ballantine Publishing Group, 1998), p. 103.

26. Dr. Joel Robbins, *Health Through Nutrition: How To Gain Health and Vitality Now* (Tulsa, OK: Vitality Unlimited), pp. 30-31.

27. Linda Page, N.D., Ph.D. *Stress and Energy,* (Carmel Valley, CA: Traditional Wisdom, Inc., 1999), p. 66.

28. Dr. Bruce West, *Health Alert,* Monterey, CA: 2001, Volume 18, Issue 6, pp. 1-2.

29. Ibid.

30. Dr. Bernard Jensen, *Tissue Cleansing Through Bowel Management* (Escondido, CA: Bernard Jensen, 1981), p. 51.

31. Ibid., p. 27.

32. Ibid., p. 28.

33. Lindsay Duncan, p. 2.

34. Patrick Quillin, Ph.D., *Beating Cancer With Nutrition* (Tulsa, OK: The Nutrition Times Press, Inc., 1994), p. 119.

35. DeAnn Liska and Dan Lukaczer, "Gut Restoration and Chronic Disease," *Journal of the American Nutraceutical Association* (JANA), Fall 2002, Vol. 5, No. 4, p. 23.

36. Ibid.

37. Ibid.

38. Anderson, KE, Kappas A, "Dietary Regulation of Cytochrome P450," *Annu Rev Nutr* 1991:11:141-67.

39. Boyd EM, Chen CP, "Lindane Toxicity and Protein-Deficient Diet." *Arch Environ Health* 1968;17:156-63.

40. Anderson, KE, Kappas A, "Dietary Regulation of Cytochrome P450," *Annu Rev Nutr* 1991:11:141-67.

41. Brodie, MJ et al., "Drug Metabolism in White Vegetarians," *Br J Clin Pharmacology* 1980;9:523-25.

42. Standard Process Purification Programs. A patient guide to purification and weight management. L2605. Standard Process. Palmyra, WI. 2003.

43. Dr. Joel Fuhrman *Fasting and Eating for Health*, (New York, NY: St. Martins Press, 1995), p. 14.

44. Standard Process Purification Programs. A patient guide to purification and weight management. L2605. Standard Process. Palmyra, WI. 2003.

I have made every effort possible to check the accuracy of material quoted. If there is any question, or a possible mistake in quoting of any material, necessary changes will be made in future printings.

Index

T

U-V

W

X-Y-Z

Order Form

Please Print

Name _____

Address _____

City _____ State _____ Zip _____

Phone _____

E-mail _____

METHOD OF PAYMENT

Check _____ Credit Card: Visa_____ Mastercard_____

Card number _____ Exp. date_____

Authorization Signature _____

ITEM	QTY	PRICE
Why Can't I Lose Weight? ($17.95)		
Why Can't I Lose Weight Cookbook ($17.95)		
Why Can't I Stay Motivated? ($14.95)		
Why Am I So Grumpy, Dopey and Sleepy? ($11.95)		
Why Am I So Wacky? ($11.95)		
Why Eat Like Jesus Ate? ($11.95)		
Why Do I Need Whole Food Supplements? ($9.95)		
Why Do I Feel So Lousy? ($9.95)		
Why Do I Really Need Herbs? ($9.95)		
Subtotal		
Shipping & Handling Add 15%		
(Add 8% if resident of OK) Tax		
Total		

Send check or money order to:

Life Design Nutrition

Lorrie Medford, CN

PO Box 54007

Tulsa, OK 74155

918-664-4483

918-664-0300 (fax)

Toll-free 1-877-716-LIFE (5433)

E-mail orders: orders@lifedesignnutrition.com

www.lifedesignnutrition.com

About the Author

Author and motivational speaker, Lorrie Medford has a B.A. in Communications and is a licensed Certified Nutritionist from The American Health Science University. She also holds certification as a personal trainer from The International Sports Science Association (ISSA). She is a member of the Oklahoma Speakers Association and also serves on the Advisory Board for Standard Process, Inc.

In addition to writing this book, she has also written *Why Can't I Stay Motivated?*, *Why Can't I Lose Weight?*, *Why Can't I Lose Weight Cookbook*, *Why Do I Need Whole-Food Supplements?*, *Why Am I So Grumpy, Dopey and Sleepy?*, and *Why Am I So Wacky?*

A health researcher and journalist, Lorrie has studied nutrition, whole-foods cooking, herbs, health, fitness, and motivation for more than 20 years. Lorrie taught her weight-loss class at a local junior college and through her own business for more than 10 years, and has taught natural foods cooking classes in Spokane, Washington and Tulsa, Oklahoma for 5 years.

She shares her knowledge in her seminars, and through her thriving nutritional consultation practice, *Life Design Nutrition,* in Tulsa, Oklahoma.

Lorrie has a rich history of community involvement teaching nutrition and is a sought-after speaker for civic groups, churches, hospitals, and wellness organizations. She is uniquely qualified to write about health and fitness. Lorrie knows what it's like to be a *cranky calorie counter* obsessed with foods, dieting, and striving to be thin. After struggling with her weight for many years, Lorrie lost more than 35 pounds and has kept it off for more than eighteen years.